全国高等医药院校药学类实验教材

生药学实验

（第三版）

主　编　殷　军

副主编　王　东

编　者　（以姓氏笔画为序）

王　东　代英辉　吕重宁

刘志惠　殷　军　韩　娜

中国健康传媒集团

中国医药科技出版社

内 容 提 要

本书为"全国高等医药院校药学类实验教材"之一，是依据高等医药院校生药学教学大纲编写，为适应教育国际化的要求，增加了英文对照内容，以便于学生在阅读英文文献、撰写英文论文时参考。全书分为实验技术和实验内容两部分。在实验技术部分中主要论述了生药学实验中常用的显微、理化鉴别及 DNA 分子鉴别实验的方法和注意事项；在实验内容部分为了让学生更好地掌握生药鉴别的共性，按照药用部位分类收载了 20 个实验，基本涵盖了生药学研究的各个方面，尤其是加入了开发性实验（药材标准的制定）、自我测试实验（未知生药粉末的鉴别）以及应用本领域新技术的实验（生药川芎的 HPLC 指纹图谱分析、高特异性 PCR 法鉴定生药蕲蛇），同时还设置了药用植物园和标本室的实习，因此具有很好的适教性和较高的参考价值。

本书可供高等医药院校相关专业实验教学（留学生教学）使用，也可供行业培训使用。

图书在版编目（CIP）数据

生药学实验/殷军主编 . —3 版 . —北京：中国医药科技出版社，2019.8

全国高等医药院校药学类实验教材

ISBN 978 – 7 – 5214 – 1285 – 7

Ⅰ. ①生… Ⅱ. ①殷… Ⅲ. ①生药学 – 实验 – 医学院校 – 教材 Ⅳ. ①R93 – 33

中国版本图书馆 CIP 数据核字（2019）第 161459 号

美术编辑　陈君杞

版式设计　郭小平

出版　**中国健康传媒集团** | 中国医药科技出版社

地址　北京市海淀区文慧园北路甲 22 号

邮编　100082

电话　发行：010 – 62227427　邮购：010 – 62236938

网址　www. cmstp. com

规格　787 × 1092mm $\frac{1}{16}$

印张　10 $\frac{1}{4}$

字数　212 千字

初版　2006 年 3 月第 1 版

版次　2019 年 8 月第 3 版

印次　2019 年 8 月第 1 次印刷

印刷　三河市腾飞印务有限公司

经销　全国各地新华书店

书号　ISBN 978 – 7 – 5214 – 1285 – 7

定价　**29. 00 元**

获取新书信息、投稿、为图书纠错，请扫码联系我们。

前　言

　　本书为"全国高等医药院校药学类实验教材之"一，是依据高等医药院校生药学教学大纲编写而成。本书是高等医药院校药学、中药学专业本科专用实验教材，还可应用于留学生教学使用。

　　全书分为实验技术和实验内容两部分。在实验技术部分中主要论述了生药学实验中常用的显微、理化鉴别及 DNA 分子实验鉴别的方法和注意事项。实验内容部分中按药用部位分类收载了 20 个实验，基本涵盖了所有生药学研究的内容，尤其是加入了开放性实验（实验十七　药材标准的制定）和自我测试实验（实验十六　未知生药粉末的鉴定），力求改变学生照单抓药的实验习惯，增强自主实验的能力。为适应生药学发展的需要，本书还收录了生药的指纹图谱分析（实验十八）和用 DNA 分子标记技术鉴别来自不同产地的生药（实验十九），并在实验中详细注明了原理、方法和程序。如果没有条件开展这些实验，也可用教师或图像演示实验代替。为弥补某些院校药学专业不设药用植物学课程的缺憾，本书加设了在药用植物园和标本室的实习（实验二十）。本版教材修订了上版书中过时内容和错误之处，如总论中显微镜使用部分，实验四及实验六；增添了新的内容：总论中加入质谱联用方法，生药的 DNA 分子鉴定方法，实验十一中加入动物类生药鹿茸的鉴定，实验十二中增添了蟾酥中脂蟾毒配基、华蟾酥毒基 HPLC 含量测定方法，实验十五中增加了多糖类和黄酮类的鉴别方法，实验十八中增加了川芎中阿魏酸的含量测定方法，实验十九中应用 PCR－RFLP 法鉴定生药川贝母；调整了原书中部分实验内容的章节顺序，如上版书中实验五中薄荷的鉴定，因其药用部位为全草类，调整至实验九等。

　　本书是由沈阳药科大学生药学教研室教师编写的。中文部分第一章第五节由韩娜教授和王东副教授共同编写，第二章实验二、三、八由韩娜副教授编写；实验一、十、十八、十九由王东副教授编写；实验四、五、六及七由刘志惠讲师编写；实验九、十一、十二、十三由代英辉讲师编写，实验十四、十五、十六由吕重宁讲师编写，其余部分由殷军教授编写并统编全书，韩娜副教授、于青讲师协助了部分校正工作。全文的英文翻译除实验十八、十九由王东副教授翻译外，其他部分均由殷军教授完成。本校硕士研究生王笑康参加了部分编译工作，日本富山医科药科大学外籍教师 Faisal Haider 先生对本书的英文内容进行了校订，在此表示谢意。本书可供高等医药院校相关专业实验教学（留学生教学）使用，也可供行业培训使用。

　　在编写过程中，由于时间仓促，水平有限，难免存在错误和疏漏之处，敬请批评指正。

编　者
2019 年 6 月

目录

contents

实验室规则

1. 遵守实验时间，不得无故缺席或迟到、早退，如中途有事离开实验室，必须征得老师同意。

2. 每次实验内容事先应充分预习，并备好应携带的物品及有关参考资料（包括实验指导及教材）。

3. 爱护实验室内的一切公共财物。使用显微镜必须严格遵守操作规程，不得随意拆动。每次使用完毕要擦拭干净，妥善放置。如有损坏，应及时主动报告，并明确责任。

4. 爱护实验室内所准备的标本、样品（药材、显微切片等），观察后必须归还，不得损坏或私自携带出室外。

5. 实验室内应保持安静，严禁吸烟、随便说笑。

6. 有机溶剂、腐蚀性液体必须倒在废液缸内，不得倒入下水道。

7. 取用公共仪器、试剂、药材应及时放回原位，不得移到个人台面上使用。

8. 实验过程中必须遵守防火和防中毒的一切规则，杜绝一切可能发生的危险隐患。

9. 实验结束后，桌面清洗干净，洗净仪器、用具，归还原位。将报告交给指导老师检查后，方可离开实验室。

Regulations of Laboratory

1. Be punctual, do not be absent, late or leave early without reasons. If you want to leave the laboratory during the experiment, you must get the teacher's permission.

2. Thoroughly preview the contents of experiment in advance and get ready for the materials and reference books requested (including experiment guidance and textbook).

3. Take care of all the materials in the laboratory. When using the microscope, you must comply with the operating regulations strictly, and should handle the microscope carefully. Always after using, make it clean and place it correctly. If it is damaged, inform your teacher immediately and make yourself clear.

4. Take care of the specimen, showpiece (medicinal materials, slices, etc), and return after observation. Do not make any damage or take it out.

5. Be quiet and do not speak or laugh loudly. Smoking is forbidden.

6. Pour organic solvent and caustic liquid into waste jar. Do not pour it into drains.

7. Return the public apparatus, reagents andmaterials to the originl place; do not move them to your individual table.

8. Obey all the fireproofing and toxicosis rules during the experiment to stop all dangerous hidden troubles.

9. Once the experiment is over, clean up all the used tools, including your tabletop, instruments and appliance and put them back. You should not leave until you handover to your supervisor your experimental report.

第一章　实验技术

　　生药的鉴别包括基原、性状、显微、理化、DNA 分子鉴定等，其中技术要求较高的是生药的显微、理化鉴定和 DNA 分子鉴定。生药学实验的重点也是指导学生掌握生药的显微和理化鉴定的方法。生药的显微鉴定主要涉及到了显微镜的使用和生药显微标本的制作。生药的理化鉴定主要包括生药中主要化学成分的定性分析、微量升华法分析、荧光分析法分析、分光光度法和色谱法分析。DNA 分子鉴定主要包括限制性片段长度多态性（RFLP）标记技术、随机扩增 DNA 多态性（RAPD）标记技术、扩增酶切片段多态性（AFLP）标记技术、简单重复序列区间（ISSR）标记技术、DNA 条形码技术等。下面就生药学实验中常用到的显微镜的使用、生药显微标本的制作、显微绘图法、显微化学鉴定、微量升华法、荧光法、分光光度法、色谱法及质谱联用技术、生药的 DNA 分子鉴定做详细论述。

Chapter One Experimental Techniques

　　To identify crude drug usually four traditional methods are used, which are original plant, description of morphous, microscopic characteristics, physical and chemical identifying methods. DNA molecular identification methods. Among them the later two methods need more technological skills. The point of our experiments is to guide students to learn microscopic characteristics and physical and chemical identifying methods. The microscopic identification mainly refers to identifying crude drugs by using a microscope and preparation of specimen. Physical and chemical identifying methods mainly include qualitative assay, microsublimation, fluorometric analysis, spectrophotometry and chromatography of main chemical compositions in crude drugs. DNA molecular identification methods includes Restriction fragment length polymorphism (RFLP) labeling technology, Random amplified DNA polymorphism (RAPD) marker technology, Amplification fragment polymorphism (AFLP) labeling technology, Inter – Simple Sequence Repeat (ISSR) Labeling Technology and DNA barcoding. The following are detailed discussion about usage of microscope, preparation of specimens, microscopic chartography, microscopic chemical identification, microsublimation, fluorometric method, spectrophotometry, chromatography and DNA molecular identification methods.

第一节 显微镜的构造及使用注意事项

一、显微镜的类型

显微镜是研究生物的细胞结构、组织特征和器官构造重要的且不可替代的仪器，它主要包括以下种类。

1. 光学显微镜 以可见光作光源，用玻璃制作透镜的显微镜。可分为单式显微镜和复式显微镜。复式显微镜结构复杂，至少由两组以上透镜组成，是植物形态解剖实验最常用的显微镜，其有效放大倍数可达 1250 倍，最高分辨力为 0.2 μm。除一般显微实验使用的普通生物显微镜外，重要的可供研究用的还有暗视野显微镜，相差显微镜和荧光显微镜。

2. 电子显微镜 是使用电子束为光源的显微镜，它以特殊的电极和磁极作为透镜代替玻璃透镜，能分辨相距 2Å（1 Å = 1/10000 mm）左右的物体，放大倍数可达 80 万 ~ 120 万倍，其分辨力比光学显微镜大 1000 倍，是观察超微结构的重要精密仪器。

二、显微镜的构造

显微镜的基本构造包括保证成像的光学系统和用以装置光学系统的机械部分，如图 1 - 1。

1. 机械部分

（1）镜座 显微镜的底座，支持全部镜体，使显微镜放置稳固。

（2）镜柱 镜座上面直立的短柱，支持镜体上部的各部分。

（3）镜臂 弯曲如臂，下连镜柱，上连镜筒，为取放镜体时手握的部分。

（4）镜筒 为显微镜上部圆柱中空的长筒，其上端置目镜，下端与目镜转换器相连。转换器下的镜筒能保护成像的光路和亮度。

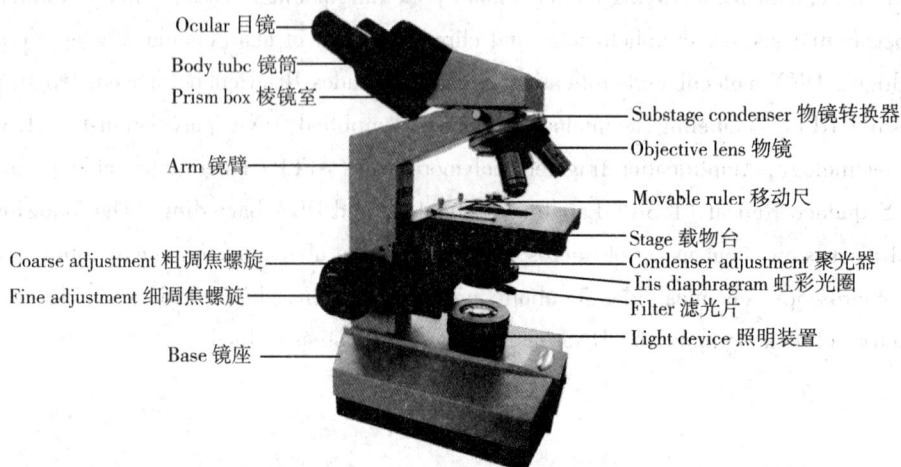

Ocular 目镜
Body tube 镜筒
Prism box 棱镜室
Arm 镜臂
Coarse adjustment 粗调焦螺旋
Fine adjustment 细调焦螺旋
Base 镜座

Substage condenser 物镜转换器
Objective lens 物镜
Movable ruler 移动尺
Stage 载物台
Condenser adjustment 聚光器
Iris diaphragm 虹彩光圈
Filter 滤光片
Light device 照明装置

图 1 - 1 双筒显微镜的构造

（5）物镜转换器　接于镜筒下端的圆盘，可自由转动。盘上有3~4个安装物镜的螺旋孔。当旋转转换器时，物镜即可固定在使用的位置上，保证物镜与目镜的光线合轴。

（6）载物台（镜台）　为放置玻片标本的平台，中央有一通光孔。上面装有机械移动器，一方面可固定玻片标本，同时可以向前后左右移动，便于观察，有的上面还装有游尺。

（7）调焦装置　用以调节物镜和标本之间的距离，使得到清晰的图像。在镜柱两侧有粗、细调焦螺旋各一对，旋转时可使载物台上升或下降，大的一对为粗调焦螺旋，旋转一周可使载物台移动2 mm左右，小的一对为细调焦螺旋，旋转一周可使载物台移动约0.1 mm。

2. 光学部分　由成像系统和照明系统组成。成像系统包括物镜和目镜，照明系统包括反光镜和聚光器。

（1）物镜　安装在镜筒下端的物镜转换器上，可分低倍、高倍和油浸物镜3种。物镜可将被检物体作第一次放大，一般其上均刻有放大倍数和数值孔径（N.A），即镜口率，如国产XSP—3C型显微镜有以下3种（表1-1）。

表1-1　XSP—3C型显微镜

物镜倍数	数值孔径（N.A）	工作距离（mm）
4×	0.1	37.5
10×	0.25	7.31
40×	0.65	0.63

工作距离是指物镜最下面透镜的表面与盖玻片上表面间的距离。物镜的放大倍数愈高，它的工作距离愈小（表1-1）。所以使用时要特别注意。

（2）目镜　安装在镜筒上端，可将物镜所成的像进一步放大。其上刻有放大倍数，如5×、10×、16×等。

（3）反光镜　是个圆形的两面镜。一面是平面镜，能反光；另一面是凹面镜，兼有反光和汇集光线的作用。反光镜具有转动关节，可作各种方向的翻转。将光线反射在聚光器上。

（4）聚光器　装于载物台下，由聚光镜和虹彩光圈等组成，它可将平行的光线汇集成束，集中于一点以增强被检物体的照明。

（5）虹彩光圈　装在聚光器内，拨动操作柄，可调节光圈大小，控制通光量。

三、显微镜的使用方法

1. 取镜和放镜　按固定编号从镜柜上取出显微镜。取镜时应右手握住镜臂，左手平托镜座，保持镜体直立，严禁用单手提着显微镜走动，防止螺旋脱扣。放置桌上时，一般应放在座位的左侧，距桌边约10~15 cm处，以便观察和防止掉落。

2. 低倍镜的使用　观察任何标本，都必须先用低倍镜，因低倍镜的视野大，容易发现目标和确定要观察的部位。

（1）放置切片　降低载物台，把玻片标本放在载物台中央，使材料正对通光孔。

然后用移动器固定住载玻片的两端。

（2）调整焦点　两眼从侧面注视物镜，并慢慢按顺时针方向转动粗调焦螺旋，使载物台徐徐上升至物镜离玻片约 5 mm 处。用双眼注视镜筒内，同时按逆时针方向转动粗调焦螺旋使载物台下降，直到看到清晰的物像为止（注意不可在调焦时边观察边上升载物台，否则会使物镜和玻片触碰，压碎玻片，损伤物镜）。如一次看不到，应重新检查材料是否放在光轴线上，重新移正材料，再重复上述操作过程直至物像出现和清晰为止。

为了使物像更加清晰，此时可轻微转动细调焦螺旋使之最清晰。当细调焦螺旋向上或向下转不动时，即表明已达极限，切勿再硬拧，而应重新调节粗调焦螺旋，拉开物镜与标本间的距离，再反拧细调焦螺旋，约 10 圈左右，（一般可动范围为 20 圈）。有的显微镜可把微调基线拧到指示微调范围的二条白线之间，再重新调整焦点至物像清晰为止。

（3）低倍镜下的观察　焦点调好后，可根据需要，移动玻片使要观察的部分在最佳位置上。找到物像后，还要根据材料的厚薄、颜色、成像反差强弱是否合适等再调节，如视野太亮，可缩小虹彩光圈，反之则开大光圈。

3. 高倍镜的使用

（1）选好目标　因高倍镜只能将低倍镜视野中心的一部分加以放大，故在使用高倍镜前应在低倍镜中选好目标并移至视野的中央，转动物镜转换器，把低倍物镜移开，换上高倍物镜，并使之与镜筒成一直线（因高倍镜工作距离很短，操作时要小心，防止镜头碰击玻片）。

（2）调整焦点　在正常情况下，当高倍物镜转正之后，在视野中即可见模糊物像，只要稍调动细调焦螺旋，即可见到最清晰的物像。注意高倍镜下不得调节粗调焦螺旋。

初用一台显微镜时，要注意它的高、低倍物镜是否能如上述情形很好配合，如果高倍物镜离盖玻片较远看不到物像时，则需重新调整焦点；此时应从侧面注视物镜，并小心转动粗调焦螺旋使载物台慢慢上升到高倍镜头几乎要与切片接触时为止（小心勿压碎玻片标本和损坏镜头），然后再由目镜观察，同时转动粗调焦螺旋，稍微降低载物台至见到物像后，换调细调焦螺旋，使物像更加清晰为止。

（3）调节亮度　在使用高倍镜观察时，视野变小变暗，所以要重新调节视野的亮度，此时可以放大虹彩圈或用凹面镜。

4. 显微镜使用后的整理　观察结束后，应先降低载物台，取下玻片，切忌在高倍镜头下取、放玻片！转动物镜转换器使物镜镜头与通光孔错开再升高载物台，擦净镜体，罩上防尘罩。仍用右手握住镜臂，左手平托镜体，按号放回镜柜中。

四、显微测量法

在生药的显微鉴定工作中，经常要用显微测量标尺测量所观察的微细物像的大小。测量长度的微量尺有载台量尺和目测量尺。

（1）载台量尺　为一种在载玻片中央刻有微细刻度的特制标尺。刻度全长 1 mm，精确等分为 10 大格，100 小格，所以每小格 10 μm。刻度外围有一小黑圈，以便易于找到标尺。载台量尺不作为直接测量物体长度使用。

（2）目镜量尺 放在目镜内的一种标尺，为一块直径 20～21 mm 的圆形玻璃片，上面刻着精细刻度 50～200 个。目镜标尺是直接用来测量物体大小的。还有一种网格式标尺是用来计算数目和测量面积的。

（3）细胞及细胞后含物的测量 先将目镜量尺装入目镜的铁圈上，用载台量尺标化。首先转动目镜，移动载台量尺，使两尺的刻度平行，且一端重合，再找出另一端的重合刻度，分别记录目镜量尺和载台量尺重合范围内的刻度，计算出目镜量尺每一小格在该物镜条件下的大小（μm）。例：用 5×目镜和 40×物镜，测得目镜量尺 100 格等于载台量尺的 50 格，即目镜量尺在这一组合中每格实际长度为 5 μm。测量细胞及细胞后含物时，被检物的长宽等于与之相当的目镜量尺小格数×5 μm，即得。如果目镜改变时，必须重新标化和计算。

五、显微镜使用的注意事项

（1）应随时保持清洁。机械部分可用软毛巾擦拭；光学部分的灰尘必须用镜头刷拂去，或用吹风机吹去后，再用擦镜纸轻擦。切忌用手指或其他粗糙物如纱布等擦拭，以免损坏镜面。

（2）用显微镜观察时，必须同时双眼睁开，切忌紧闭一眼。要反复训练用左眼窥镜，右眼作图。

（3）用于观察的标本必须加盖盖玻片，制作带有试剂的玻片标本时，必须两面擦干后，再放在载物台上观察。

（4）如遇部件失灵、使用困难时，不可强行转动，更不可任意拆修，应立即报告指导教师解决，以免造成损坏。

Section 1　Structure of Microscope and Announcement of Usage

1. Types of microscopes

The microscope is an important and irreplaceable instrument in research of cytoarchitecture, tissue signature and organ construction, including main types as follows.

（1）Optical microscope It is a microscope whose lensis made of glass, using visible light as light source. They are classified as single and compound types. The compound microscope with complex structure is the commonest type in plants anatomy experiments and is made up of at least two groups of lenses, with the enlargement factor of 1250 and the highest resolving power of 0.2 mm. Besides the common biological microscopes for general microscopic experiments, there are other kinds for research, such as the darkfield microscope, contrast phase microscope and fluorescence microscope.

（2）Electron microscope It is the microscope using electron beam aslight source; its lenses are made of special electrode and magnetic pole instead of glass. It can distinguish any objects away from 2Å (1Å = 1/10000 μm), and its enlargement factor can be 800 000 – 1 200 000 and resolving power is 1000 times of that of optical microscope. It is an important exquisite apparatus for ultrastructure.

2. The structure of compound microscope

The basic structure includes two parts: the optical system for imaging and the mechanical system for fixing optical system.

（1）Mechanical system

① Base   A basic unit of microscope upholds the whole lens body and makes it steady.

② Column   A short erect column on the base upholds the parts above it.

③ Arm   An arm – likepart connects the base and the body tube for holding.

④ Body tube   A long tube connecting the ocular and objective lens converter protects beam path and brightness of imaging.

⑤ Substage condenser   A disc under the column can be turned freely. There are 3 – 4 screw poles for objective lenses on it. When it is turned, the objective lens can be fixed at acertain place to make the light of objective and ocular lens on the same line.

⑥ Stage   It is a platform on which the specimen is placed. There is an opening in the center, through which light passes through. The clip on it can fix a slide and the turner under the platform can move the slide to every position. Sometimes there is a vernier on the stage.

⑦ Adjustments   A deviceis used for bringing a specimen into focus. On both sides of the pole there are coarse adjustments and fine adjustments to move the stage up and down when it is turned. The bigger ones are coarse adjustments, which can move the stage about 2 mm when they are turned a circle. The small couple is fine adjustments and the same operation makes the stage moved about 0. 1 mm.

（2）Optical system   This part is made up of imaging system and illuminating system. The imaging system contains an objective and ocular. The illuminating system contains a mirror and condenser adjustment. The microscope without mirror uses electric light.

①Objective lenses   They are setted within the substage condenser and can be classified asthe lower – power, high – power, and oil – immersion lens. They magnify a specimen primarily. Enlargement factor and numberical aperture（NA）are wroten on them generally, for example, here is some data about XSP – 3C, the domestic product.

Multiple of objective lens	Numberical aperture（NA）	Working distance（mm）
4 ×	0. 1	37. 5
10 ×	0. 25	7. 31
40 ×	0. 65	0. 63

The working distance is defined as the distance between lens surface and a specimen. The smaller the working distance is, the greater enlargement factor will be. So should be more careful in use.

② Ocular   They are assembled on top of the column and can magnify the image secondly. There are enlargement factors on them, such as $5 \times$, $10 \times$, $16 \times$, and so on.

③ Mirror　It is a two – side round mirror. One side is a plane mirror reflecting light; the other side is concave that can reflect and collect light. The turner on this mirror can turn over to various kinds of direction to reflect light on the condenser adjustment.

④ Condenser adjustment　It is assembled under the stage and is made up of a condenser and an iris diaphragm. It can collect parallel light into a beam to make a specimen bright.

⑤ Iris diaphragm　It is fixed in the condenser adjustment. We can adjust the size of the diaphragm by turning the operation bar as to control the light quantity.

3. Usage of microscope

(1) Taking and placing　Take out a microscope from cupboard with the mounting number. You must hold the arm with your right hand and support the base with your left hand to make the whole body steady and erect. You shouldn't lift a microscope with a single hand; otherwise its screw will be loosed. A microscope should be put on the left side of your seat in a distance of 10 – 15 cm from the table edge in order to observe and prevent from falling down.

(2) Usage of a low – power objective lens　Whenever you observe a specimen, you should start with the low – power objective lens. The low – power objective lens can give a wider vision field so that you can find your goal and the objected part easily.

① Fix a slide　Lower the stage, set a slide specimen right in the center of stage and make the point you want to the pore, and then fix the slide with two clips on the stage.

② Adjust the focus　Look at the objective lens sideward, slowly turn the coarse adjustments clockwise to raise the stage until the distance between the objective lens and the slide is about 5 mm. Observe the vision with your eyes and turn the coarse adjustments counterclockwise until you see the image precisely. (Don't raise the stage when observing, otherwise you may smash the objective lens and the slide). If you can't see any image, check whether your material is right on the light axis, remove it and follow the above mentioned points again till you can see your goal clearly.

In order to make the image clearer, turn the fine adjustment slightly. When the fine adjustment can't move up or down any more, it has reached its limit. Don't move it any more roughly, just readjust your coarse adjustment again, enlarge the distance between the objective and the specimen, and then turn your fine adjustment towards the other side about 10 loops (20 loops is a limit). In some microscopes the baseline of fine adjustment can be settled within the two white lines, and then the focus is adjusted to get a clear vision.

③ Test under a low – power objective lens　After the focus is achieved, you can move the slide to the best place as you want. You could also adjust focus again according to the thickness, color of your material and the contrast degree of the image after you find it. For instance, if the vision is too light, turn down the iris diaphragm, otherwise, turn it up on the contrary.

(3) Usage of a high – power objective lens

① Search for your goal　You should make your goal right in the center of the vision under the low – power objective lens before using the high – power one, because the latter only can zoom in the central vision under the former one. Then turn the low – power lens away with a high – power one instead to make sure that it holds a line with the body tube. (Take care to prevent from breaking lens or slide because of the short working distance of a high – power lens)

②Adjust the focus As the high – power lens turns right, we can see the vision vaguely. After adjusting the fine adjustment a little, we can see it clearly. You must remember that coarse adjustment should not be turned under a high – power lens.

When you use a microscope for the first time, make sure if its low and high power lens match well as above. If not, readjust your focus as following. Observe the objective sideward, ascend the coarse adjustment slightly till it is going to touch the slice (Be sure not to break either a slice or lens), and then observe it from the ocular. Lower the stage by using coarse adjustment until the image appears, and then turn fine adjustment again to make the image clearer.

③ Adjust the brightness When you turn into a high – power lens, the field of vision will be smaller and darker. Readjust the brightness of your vision by magnifying the iris diaphragm or using the concave mirror.

(4) Tidying up After your experiment, lower the stage, get the slice off, turn the condenser to leave light condenser from the pore, lift the stage again, make the whole body clean and cover the dustproof cover. Place the microscope back into the cupboard in the same way as you brought it out.

4. Microscopic measurement

When we work on microscopic identification of crude drugs, we usually use the micrometers included a stage micrometer and ocular micrometer to measure the size of minute image.

(1) Stage micrometer It is a special slide with a graduated meter at the center, which possesses 100 divisions of each 10 μm in length of 1 mm. There is a black circle surrounding the meter in order to easily find. The stage micrometer isn't used for measuring length of object directly.

(2) Ocular micrometer It is a meter on ocular, a disc slide with a diameter of 20 – 21 mm and 50 – 200 fine divisions on it. Ocular micrometer is used for measuring length of object directly. Another kind is a grid like meter used for counting number and measure area of object.

(3) Measuring of cells and their ergastic substances Put an ocular micrometer onto the iron coil of ocular, and standardize it with a stage micrometer. Turn the ocular, move the stage micrometer, make the two graduations parallel when the one end of 2 micrometers are coincidence and find the coincident graduation of another end to note the graduation numbers of 2 micrometers in superposition scope. Calculate the length of each graduation on the ocular micrometer amount to that of the stage micrometer (μm). For example: for a microscope with 5 × ocular and 10 ×objective, the length of 100 graduations on the ocular micrometer equals to that of 50 graduations on the stage micrometer, so the length of each graduation on the ocular mi-

crometer is 5 μm. When cells or their ergastic substances are measured, their size is the data which corresponded graduations multiple 5 μm. If we use different kinds of ocular, we must standardize and calculate them again.

5. Usage announcements

(1) Keep your microscope tidy all the time, wipe the mechanical part clean with a soft washcloth, and clean the ocular part with a lens – used brush or blow the dust away before you wipe it with a piece of lens – cleaned paper. Be sure not to wipe it with your hands or some other coarse things like gauze otherwise you may scrape the lens.

(2) Use both of your eyes to observe, and do not close either of them. Always be practicing to use your left eye for observing and the other for drawing.

(3) You must put a cover glass on a specimen before observing under a microscope. If you make water or other solutions over the slice, be sure to wipe both sides of the plate glass clean before you place it on the stage.

(4) If there is some part not working, don't try to turn it forcibly or even take it apart. In order to avoid more damage, you should tell your teacher.

第二节 生药显微标本的制作

在生药的显微鉴定中，样品需制成显微标本后，才可在显微镜下观察。生药的显微标本包括临时标本和永久标本。学生实验中自己动手制作的主要是临时标本，所以这里主要介绍永久标本的种类及临时标本的制作方法。

一、永久标本

(1) 徒手切片后封藏。

(2) 滑走切片后封藏　用滑走切片机进行切片。

(3) 解离组织后封藏　用化学试剂使细胞的胞间层溶解，细胞彼此分离，以便观察不同的细胞形态特征。

(4) 石蜡切片　制作永久切片最常用的方法。对不易切片的样品，利用石蜡渗入植物组织中，用旋转切片机进行切片，然后再将切片中石蜡除去。

二、临时标本的制作方法

1. **粉末制片法**　本法用于制备粉末状生药、以生药粉末制备的中成药及其原料药材粉末的显微鉴定制片法，是生药显微鉴别中最常用的制片法。一般是先将药材烘干、粉碎，过5～6号筛。取粉末适量（约半粒大米粒大小），加水（不透化，观察淀粉粒），或加水合氯醛，加热、透化，再加稀甘油（观察细胞、草酸钙结晶等后含物），或加乙醇（观察橙皮苷或菊糖团块）。

2. **表皮制片法**　本法适用于观察叶片花萼、花瓣、雄蕊以及浆果、草质茎、根茎等的表皮显微鉴定特征。较薄的材料可整体封藏，其他材料可撕取或削取表皮制作。

若为干的材料，如较薄的叶、花类生药可用冷水浸泡至能伸展、恢复原样后，用刀片在表面轻轻浅划一刀，用小镊子从切口处撕取表皮，切去带表皮下部组织的那部分表皮。若为较软的浆果类，可直接削取表皮。如较硬的则需要经软化处理。水合氯醛试液透化后，加甘油封藏。

制好的临时标本片，要求封藏剂适度，不足时，可用滴管从盖玻片的边缘滴加少许，盖玻片边缘多余的液体，可用吸水纸从玻片的一端吸去。

3. **徒手切片法** 本法是用剃刀或保险刀片把新鲜的、预先固定好的或软化的材料切成薄片，不染色或经简单染色，用水封片后观察。一般是先将材料切成 2～3 cm 的小段，坚硬的材料可用水煮、50% 乙醇－甘油（1:1）浸泡，软化后再切片。若材料过软时，则可置 70%～95% 乙醇中浸泡 20～30 分钟。切片时，左手拇指和示指夹住材料，用中指托起，材料要高于手指。将刀口放在外缘的 1/4 左右处，刀片贴切面平拉，不要担心切片太薄或不完整而将刀口向下。注意切忌来回拉锯。将切下的薄片用湿毛笔转移到盛水的培养皿中，再选最薄的切片放在载玻片上观察，也可用 0.1% 番红溶液给细胞核及木质化、栓质化的细胞壁染色后再观察。

Section 2　Preparation of Microscopic Specimens of Crude Drugs

Working on microscopic identification of the crude drugs, the samples should be made into microscopic specimens before testing under microscope. The microscopic specimens of crude drugs include temporary and permanent ones. The specimens the students prepare by themselves are mainly temporary specimens. So this section chiefly introduces the varieties of permanent specimens and the preparing methods of temporary specimens.

1. Permanent specimens

（1）Mounting after a hand section.

（2）Mounting after a sliding section　It is the method of cutting slices by a sliding microtome.

（3）Mounting a kind of dissociated tissue　It is the method of dissolving intercellular layers with chemical reagents to make the cells separated from each other, so that we can observe the morphological characteristics of various cells.

（4）Paraffin sections　It is the commonest method of making permanent slices. When the samples are not easy to cut, we can make the paraffin permeate into plant tissues and cut them by a rotary microtome, then remove the paraffin in the slices.

2. Methods for temporary specimens

（1）Mounting the powder of crude drugs　This method is applicable to prepare the specimens of crude drugs powder, the Chinese formulated products made by powder of crude drugs and raw medicinal material. It is the commonest specimen – preparing method in the microscopic identification of crude drugs. Generally dry the materials first, shatter, sieve with the No. 5 – 6 sifter. Then take some of powder, add water (to observe starch grains without permeabilizing) or permeabilize with chloral hydrate, then add dilute glycerin (to observe cells or their ergastic substances like calcium oxalate crystals) or add ethanol (to observe hesperidin or inulin).

(2) Mounting an epidermis The method is to observe microscopic identification characteristics of the epidermis of a leave blade, calyx, petal, stamen, berry, herbaceous stem and rhizome. The thinner materials can be mounted their whole body, the other thicker epidermis is needed to be torn or be cut. For the dried materials, like thinner leaves or flowers, we may soak them in cold water until they recover unfolding; score lightly on the surface with blade, take a piece of epidermis from cutting and remove the diachyma part. For a softer berry, we may pare its epidermis directly. As to the hard ones, we may process them by softening. Permeabilize with chloral hydrate and mount with glycerin.

(3) Preparing method for a hand section This method is to cut the fresh, fixed or softened drug materials into slides with blade or razor, nonstaining or being dyed simply, to observe after mounting with water. Generally cut the materials into 2 – 3 cm long portions; for the harder materials, we may boil or soak them with 50% ethanol – glycerin (1:1); for the too soft materials, we may soak them with 70% – 95% ethanol for 20 – 30 min. When cutting, clamp the material with thumb and forefinger of your left hand, supporting with your middle finger to make the material high than your fingers. Put the blade on the 1/4 portion of outer margin, move the blade parallel to a tangent plane. Don't worry about the cut slice will be too thin and to make the blade downward. Never move the blade back and forth. Move the cut slices into the culture dish and put some water on them with writing brush. Choose the thinnest one to put on a glass slide to observe; or you can dye the cell nucleus, the lignified and suberized cell wall with 0.1% safranine solution to observe.

第三节 绘图方法与要求

绘图是实验报告的重要内容之一，正确地绘出生药的外观图及组织、粉末的显微结构图，不仅可以加深对植物形态和结构特征的认识，还可以帮助养成认真的观察习惯，是学习生药的性状和显微结构特征必须掌握的基本技能。

由于学生实验时间较短，在实验课上将组织中大量的细胞全面地绘出是不可能的，因而可要求学生细致地画出1/4~1/2，剩余部分画出轮廓，细致部分略去。

一、注意事项

（1）首先要注意准确性和代表性。要认真观察要画的标本或切片，选择正常的、典型的、有代表性的材料或部分，正确理解各部分的特征，才能保证所绘的图像是准确的，有代表意义的。

（2）实验题目写在绘图纸的上方，图题和所用材料的名称、部分标在图的下方，并注明放大倍数。图注用平行线引出在图的右侧，并用铅笔正楷书写。

（3）画图前先构图。应按实验指导要求的绘图的数量和内容，在绘图纸上先安排好各图的位置和相关部分的比例，并留出书写图题和注释的部分。

（4）绘图时，首先画轮廓，即用 HB 铅笔轻轻在绘图纸上勾画出图形的轮廓，然后用 2H 铅笔描出细致部位，线条要粗细均匀，光滑清晰，接头处无分叉，切忌重复描画（铅笔尖要细，切忌变粗时使用）。

（5）植物图常用圆点的疏密表示明暗和颜色的深浅，圆点应圆而整齐，大小均匀，切忌用涂抹阴影的方法代替圆点。对晶体类等需要显示立体结构的，应运用立体几何知识绘图，被遮盖的部分或下层，引用虚线表示，表示深颜色时用加点方法。

二、生药绘图的方法

1. 外观图的描画法　有以下 3 种：写生实物法、放大照片描绘法及格子玻璃板放大法。其中第 3 种方法即格子玻璃板放大法，是指将画有格子的适当大小的玻璃板（每个格子为 5 mm × 5 mm）放在生药上，一边观察每个格子中生药的形态，一边在用铅笔轻画出格子的绘图纸上（每 3 个格为 10 mm × 10 mm）勾画出生药的轮廓及特征图，最后将细致部分描画。制版时还必须将半透明的硫酸纸覆在已绘好的底图上，用绘图铅笔描成墨线图。

2. 组织、粉末镜检图描画法　生药的组织特征图可分为组织简图和组织详图。

绘制植物的显微结构简图时，常用一些通用的画线方式和符号来表示各种不同的组织，如图 1-2 所示。

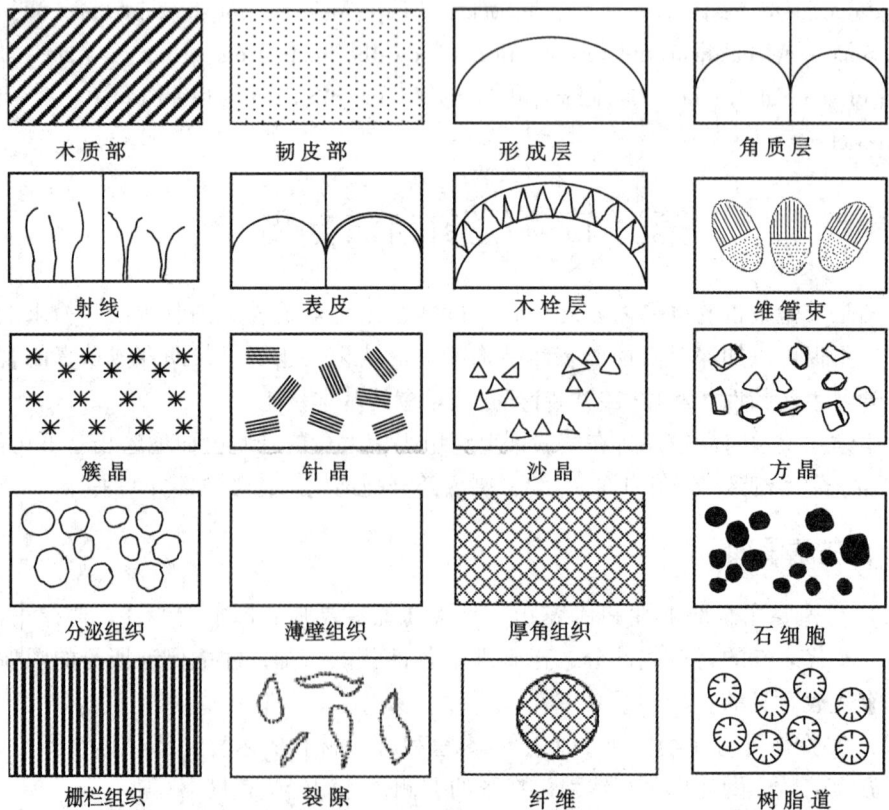

图 1-2　植物组织、后含物简图常用符号

　　组织详图（包括解离组织图和生药粉末特征图）是表明生药组织中各种细胞及后含物的形状及排列方式的。有横切面、纵切面、表面观 3 种图。在此类图中，不必画出所有的观察到的细胞，一般只画十几个到几十个有代表性的、能说明问题的细胞即可。但每个细胞的形状、壁厚、纹孔、层纹等细部，都要画准确。

　　（1）徒手绘图法　将绘图纸放在显微镜右侧，左眼观察显微镜内物像。选择好具有特征性的组织或后含物，用 HB 铅笔将物像轻轻画在绘图纸上，再仔细观察物像，反复对照修改直至满意，最后用 2H 铅笔稍重地勾画一遍。如果要制作发表论文或出版书籍用的墨线图时，将半透明的硫酸纸置于绘好的铅笔图上，用特制的绘图笔照底图描绘即可。方法简便易行，但绘图易在形状、各部分的比例方面失真。

　　（2）显微绘图器绘图法　常用的显微绘图器包括：阿贝氏描绘器、描绘棱镜、目镜及投影式描绘器。

　　阿贝氏描绘器是一个由两个棱镜构成的棱镜筒和一个平面反射镜构成的装置，将棱镜筒接在显微镜的目镜后，通过调节反射镜的位置，使视野中组织构造和笔尖、绘图纸同时清晰可见，即可用铅笔依样描绘，再用墨线笔重描。

　　描绘棱镜是将棱镜接在显微镜目镜上，而描绘目镜是用带有目镜的棱镜替换掉显微镜的目镜。

　　在使用显微描绘器描绘生药的组织构造或粉末的显微特征时需注意以下问题：① 绘图板面要调节到与描绘器的反射棱镜外侧镜面平行，才可保证物像图各部位的放大倍数都相同，避免图形失真；② 物像超过一个视野时，画完一个视野，要移动这个视野前，需记忆 2~3 个明显的标志，以便移动后物像与图像能准确地衔接；③ 为了消除物镜的球面效应使物像失真的现象，描绘时应将目的物移到视野的中央，且每次移动的最大范围不超过 2/3 个视野。

Section 3　Drawing Methods and Requests

Drawing is one of the important parts in an experimental report. A correct outside picture and microstructure picture of tissue, powder of crude drugs can not only impress us the plant morphous and tissue structure, but also help us to get used to careful observation; it is a basic skill of learning pharmacognosy.

It is impossible to draw all the tissue because of the limited time of the students' experiment. So the students can draw 1/2 – 1/4 of whole part in detail and draw the outline of the rest.

1. Announcement

（1）Pay attention to the accuracy and typicality. Observe a target specimen or slice carefully, choose a normal, typical and representative part, comprehend the characteristics of each portion correctly to ensure a picture drawing to be precise and representative.

（2）Write the experiment title in the head of your drafting paper, drawing headings and materials names, used part and the magnification below your chart; the annotation in penciled regular script, should be placed on the right side of picture, connected to annotated parts by parallel lines.

(3) Composition of a picture before drawing. Arrange the positions and correlating proportions of all figures on your drafting paper according to the required quantity and contents, and set aside the space of signs and remarks.

(4) Draw the outline first. Draw the outline of a picture on a drafting paper with a HB pencil, then draw the fine part with a 2H pencil; lines in uniform thickness should be smooth and clear, without furcations at joints; never draw repeatedly (the pencil point should be acute but coarsened).

(5) The sparse or dense dots use to indicate the brightness or darkness; the dots should be round and neat with a uniform size; never use painting shade instead of dots. For the crystals with stereochemical structure, make use of your knowledge of solid geometry to indicate the covered parts of underlayers with dash lines, to show dark color with dotting.

2. Drawing methods of crude drugs

(1) Delineating methods of outside drawing　Includes the following three methods: to paint from life, to portray a macrophotograph and to enlarge with grid glass. The third method is done by the following process: put a proper glass plate drawn with grids (each grid is 5 mm × 5 mm) on the material, observe the appearance of drugs in each grid meanwhile draw the outline and characteristics on a paper with grids by a pencil accordingly (the size of each three grids is 10 mm × 10 mm), then draw the fine part. For publish, copy the foundation picture with an ink pen on a piece of semitransparent vegetable parchment.

(2) Drawing methods of tissue and powder in testing under microscope　Tissue characteristics drawings include tissue block – diagram and detail drawing.

Here are some general scribings and symbols to indicate the different tissues in your block – diagram.

A detail drawing (including a drawing of dissociated tissue and powder characteristics) is to indicate the shape and arrangement of all kinds of cells and their ergastic substance in plant tissues. It includes that of a cross section, longitudinal section and surface appearance. It is not necessary to draw all the cells observed, but draw the dozen to decades of representative cells, and you need to draw the shape, wall thickness, pit and striation of each cell clearly.

① Unarmed drawing　Place a piece of drafting paper on the right of a microscope and observe the image with the left eye. Choose the characteristic tissues and ergastic substances, draw lightly on the paper with a HB pencil, observe the image carefully, modify repeatedly until you are satisfied, and then delineate again with 2H pencil. For publish, copy the foundation picture by covering a piece of semitransparent vegetable parchment on the drawn paper with an ink pen. However, this is a convenient and easy way but with shortcoming of distortion in shape and proportion.

② Drawing with pantographies　The common pantographies include Abbe's drawing apparatus, delineated prism, delineated ocular and projection plotter.

Abbe's drawing apparatus is made up of a prism tube with two prisms and 1 plane reflector. Connect the prism tube to ocular lens, modify the position of the reflector to make the tissue structure, pen point and paper clear in the eyesight, and then delineate with pencil and copy with darker ink lines.

Delineated prism is to connect a prism to ocular lens and a delineated ocular is to replace an ocular lens by prism with ocular lens.

The announcements of drawing tissue structure and powder characteristic with a drawing prism:

Ⅰ. A drawing board should be adjusted to be parallel to the outside reflector to ensure the same magnifying times of every part of picture as that of the observed image with a microscope.

Ⅱ. If the image exceeds eyeshot, you should memorize two or three obvious symbols before you move to the next visual field in order to that the following image can link up.

Ⅲ. In order to eliminate the distortion caused by the sphere effect, you should make the target in the center of your eyeshot; the movement range should not exceed 2/3 of your eyeshot.

第四节　生药的理化鉴定及质量分析

理化鉴定是通过物理和化学的方法，对生药（及其制剂）中所含主要成分或有效成分进行定性和定量分析，根据定性和定量分析结果，鉴定生药真伪优劣的一种方法。

一、化学成分的定性分析

有些化学试剂能与生药中的化学成分产生特殊的颜色或沉淀，用来鉴定生药中含有哪一类成分（参见人民卫生出版社蔡少青主编《生药学》教材第2章生药的化学成分）。

二、生药的显微化学反应

兼用显微鉴定和理化鉴定两种方法。一般是将生药的粉末、徒手切片或浸出液少量，置载玻片上，滴加适宜的化学试剂制成临时切片，在显微镜下观察所产生的沉淀、结晶、气泡、溶解、颜色变化等现象，以便确定细胞壁的组成、细胞后含物的性质、某种成分在生药组织中的分布，从而鉴别生药。其方法很多，下面仅介绍几种。

（一）细胞壁的组成

1. **木质化细胞壁**　一般取新鲜植物材料的切片置载玻片上，先加40%盐酸1~2滴，3~5分钟后，待材料被盐酸浸透，再加5%间苯三酚乙醇溶液，含有木质素的细胞壁就变为樱红色或紫红色。导管、管胞、纤维和石细胞等的细胞壁中木质素丰富，因此它们的颜色反应十分明显，内皮层细胞壁的凯氏点处木质素也很丰富，也常用此反应来确定它在组织切片中的存在。

2. 木栓化或角质化细胞壁 一般取新鲜植物材料作徒手切片或取粉末少量置载玻片上，加苏丹Ⅲ试液，加盖玻片后镜检，木栓化细胞壁显橘红色、红色或紫红色。

（二）细胞后含物

1. 淀粉粒 取生药粉末少量置载玻片上，加碘试液装片，淀粉粒呈蓝色或紫红色。

2. 草酸钙结晶 取生药粉末少量置载玻片上，加稀草酸装片，镜检，可见草酸钙不溶解，沿盖玻片边缘加 1～2 滴稀盐酸，草酸钙结晶溶解，不产生气泡。若用30%硫酸（V/V）装片，镜检，可见草酸钙结晶逐渐溶解，片刻后，析出硫酸钙针晶。

3. 蛋白质（糊粉粒） 细胞内贮藏的蛋白质是无生命的，呈较稳定的、无定形的、结晶状的或有固定形态的糊粉粒。糊粉粒是植物细胞中蛋白质存在的主要形式。一般取新鲜植物材料的切片置载玻片上，先加95%乙醇溶解脂肪，再加碘－碘化钾溶液，糊粉粒就变为黄色或棕色颗粒。

4. 乳汁、脂肪油、挥发油 一般取新鲜植物材料的切片置载玻片上，加苏丹Ⅲ试液，稍加热，加盖玻片后镜检，可见乳汁管中的乳汁、脂肪油、挥发油可被染成红色。

（三）显微化学定位反应

利用显微和化学方法，确定生药有效成分在生药组织构造中的部位。一般取新鲜脱水植物材料作徒手切片置载玻片上，加某种试剂后装片，镜检，观察颜色反应及存在的部位。如按上法取柴胡根横切面薄片，滴加无水乙醇和浓硫酸的等量混合液，装片，镜检，可见含柴胡皂苷的部位，最初呈黄绿色至绿色，5～10分钟后，由蓝绿色变成蓝色，此蓝色可持续1小时以上。最后变成污蓝色而消失。

三、微量升华法

有些生药中含有某些化学成分，在一定温度下具有升华的性质，微量升华就是利用这一特性，借助微量升华装置，从少量生药中获取升华物，在显微镜下观察其形状、颜色及可发生的化学反应，以鉴别生药。如大黄、何首乌中的蒽醌类成分具有升华性，温度较低时得黄色针状结晶，较高温时得黄色羽毛状结晶，高温时得黄色油滴。加碱液时结晶溶解，溶液显红色，再加盐酸溶液变黄色。斑蝥中的斑蝥素升华物为无色柱形结晶，加氢氧化钡溶液溶解，并产生针状结晶。牡丹皮中的丹皮酚升华物为无色针晶、柱状或羽状结晶，加三氯化铁试液时结晶溶解，溶液显暗紫色。

具体方法为取金属片，放置石棉板上，金属片上放一小金属圈（高度约0.8 cm），金属圈内加入生药粉末一薄层，圈上放一载玻片，用酒精灯徐徐加热数分钟，至粉末开始变焦，去火待冷，则有结晶状升华物凝集于载玻片上。将载玻片取下反转，盖上盖玻片，在显微镜下观察结晶形状，并滴加化学试液，观察其反应。必要时可用显微熔点测定器测定结晶的熔点。

四、荧光分析

利用生药中所含的某些化学成分，在紫外光或自然光下能产生一定颜色荧光的性质，是鉴定生药的一种简易方法。通常可直接取生药饮片、粉末或用其浸出液，置暗处，用荧光分析仪照射进行观察。例如黄连饮片显金黄色荧光；大黄粉末显深棕色荧光；秦皮的水浸液显天蓝色荧光等。

　　某些生药本身不产生荧光，但以酸或碱处理或经其他化学方法处理后，可使某些成分在紫外光下变为可见色彩。例如芦荟水溶液本无荧光，但与硼砂共热，所含芦荟素即起反应显黄绿色荧光。根据荧光的强弱，可用荧光分析仪进行生药的定量分析。有些生药表面附有地衣或真菌，也可能有荧光出现。因而荧光分析还可用于检查某些生药的变质情况。

　　此外可用荧光显微镜鉴别生药，如国产沉香粉末显海蓝色至灰绿色，而进口沉香粉末显绿色至枯绿色。

五、分光光度法

　　分光光度法是通过测定被测物质在特定波长处或一定波长范围内的光吸收度，对该物质进行定性和定量分析的方法。常用分光光度法如表 1 - 2 所示。

表 1 - 2　分光光度法测定范围

波长	光区	测定仪器
200～400 nm	紫外	紫外分光光度计
400～760 nm	可见	可见分光光度计或比色计
2.5～25 mm	红外	红外分光光度计
（波数 4000～400 cm^{-1}）		原子吸收分光光度计

　　单色光辐射穿过被测物质溶液时，被该物质吸收的量与该物质的浓度和液层的厚度（光路长度）成正比，其关系式为：

$$A = \lg\ (1/T)\ = Ecl \qquad\qquad (1-1)$$

　　式中，A—吸光度；

　　　　　T—透光率；

　　　　　E—吸收系数（$E_{1\,cm}^{1\%}$），其物理意义为当溶液浓度为 1%（g/ml），液层厚度为 1 cm 时的吸光度数值；

　　　　　c—100 ml 溶液中所含被测物质的质量（g，按干燥品或无水物计算）；

　　　　　l—液层厚度（cm）。

　　物质对光的吸收波长及吸收系数是该物质的物理常数。当已知某纯物质在一定条件下的吸收系数后，可用同样条件将含有此物质的供试品配成溶液，测其吸光度，即可由上式计算出供试品中该物质含量。

　　在可见光区，除某些物质对光有吸收外，很多物质本身并没有吸收，但可在一定条件下加入显色试剂或经过处理使其显色后再测定，故又称比色分析。由于显色时，影响呈色深浅的因素较多，且常使用单色光纯度较差的仪器，故测定时应用标准品或对照品同时操作。

（一）紫外分光度法

　　1. 仪器的校正和检定　由于温度变化对机械部分的影响，仪器波长经常会略有变动，因此除定期对所用仪器进行全面校正外，还应于测定前校正测定波长。常用汞灯中较强谱线 237.83 nm、253.65 nm、275.28 nm、296.73 nm、313.16 nm、334.15 nm、365.02 nm、404.66 nm、435.8 nm、546.07 nm 与 576.96 nm，或用仪器中氘灯的 486.02 nm 与 656.10 nm 谱线进行校正，钬玻璃在 279.4 nm、287.5 nm、333.7 nm、360.9 nm、418.5 nm、460.0 nm、484.5 nm、532.6 nm 与 637.5 nm 波长处有尖锐吸收峰，也可作波长校正用，但因来源不同会有微小的差别，使用时应注意。

吸光度准确度检定：可用重铬酸钾溶液。取在 120℃ 下干燥至恒重的基准重铬酸钾约 60 mg，精密称定，用 0.005mol/L 硫酸溶液溶解并稀释至 1000 ml，在规定波长处测定并计算其吸收系数，并与规定吸收系数比较，如表 1-3，相对标准偏差应在 1% 以内。

表 1-3　吸光度准确度检定（重铬酸钾溶液）

波长（nm）	235（最小）	257（最大）	313（最小）	350（最小）
吸收系数 $E_{1\,cm}^{1\%}$	124.5	144.0	48.62	106.6

杂散光检查：可按表 1-4 的试剂和浓度，配制成水溶液，置 1 cm 石英吸收池中，在规定波长处测定透光率，应符合规定。

表 1-4　杂散光检查

试　剂	浓度（%，g/ml）	测定用波长（nm）	透光（%）
碘化钠	1.00	220	<0.8
亚硝酸钠	5.00	340	<0.8

2. 溶剂的要求　测定供试品之前，应先检查所用溶剂在供试品所用波长附近是否符合要求，即用 1 cm 石英吸收池盛溶剂，以空气为空白（即空白光路中不置任何物质）测定其吸光度。溶剂和吸收池的吸光度，在 220～240 nm 范围内不得超过 0.40，在241～250 nm 范围内不得超过 0.20，在 251～300 nm 范围内不得超过 0.10，在 300 nm 以上时不得超过 0.05。

3. 测定方法　测定时除另有规定外，应以配制供试品溶液的同批溶剂为空白对照，采用 1 cm 石英吸收池，在规定的吸收峰波长 ±2 nm 以内测试几个点的吸光度，以核对供试品吸收峰波长位置是否正确，除另有规定外，吸收峰波长应在该品种项下规定的波长 ±2 nm 以内；否则应考虑该试样的真伪、纯度以及仪器波长的精确度，并以吸光度最大波长作为测定波长。一般供试品溶液吸光度读数，以在 0.3～0.7 之间误差较小。仪器的狭缝波带宽度应小于供试品吸收带宽度，否则测得的吸光度偏低；狭缝宽度的选择应以减小狭缝宽度时供试品的吸光度不再增加为准，由于吸收池和溶剂本身可能有空白吸收，因此测定供试品的吸光度后应减去空白读数，再计算含量。

用于含量测定的方法一般有以下几种。

（1）对照品比较法　分别配制供试品溶液和对照品溶液，对照品溶液中所含被测成分的含量应为供试品溶液中被测成分标示量的 100% ±10%，所用溶剂也应完全一致，在规定的波长测定供试品溶液和对照品溶液的吸光度之后，按下式计算供试品中被测溶液的浓度：

$$c_X = （A_X / A_R）c_R \tag{1-2}$$

式中，c_X—供试品溶液浓度；

A_X—供试品溶液吸光度；

c_R—对照品溶液浓度；

A_R—对照品溶液吸光度。

（2）吸收系数法　按各品种项下的方法配制供试品溶液，在规定的波长处测定其吸光度，再以该品种在规定条件下的吸收系数计算含量。用本法测定时，应注意仪器的校正和检定。

（3）计算分光光度法　采用计算分光光度法应慎重。本法有多种，当吸光度处在吸收曲线的陡然上升或下降的部位测定时，波长的微小变化可能对测定结果造成显著影响，故对照品和供试品的测试条件应尽可能一致。若测定时不用对照品，如维生素A测定法，则应在测定时对仪器进行做仔细的校正和检定。

（二）比色法

用比色法测定时，应取对照品同时操作。除另有规定外，比色法所用的空白系指用同体积溶剂代替对照品或供试品溶液，然后依次加入等量的相应试剂，并用同样方法处理。在规定的波长处测定对照品和供试品溶液的吸光度后，按紫外分光光度法测定方法对照品比较法的计算式计算供试品浓度。

当吸光度和浓度关系不成线性时，应取数份梯度量的对照品溶液，用溶剂补充至同一体积，显色后测定各份溶液的吸光度，然后以吸光度与相应的浓度绘制标准曲线，再根据供试品的吸光度在标准曲线上求出其含量。

（三）红外分光光度法

（1）仪器及其校正　傅立叶变换红外光谱仪或色散型红外分光光度计，用聚苯乙烯薄膜（厚度约为 0.05 mm）校正仪器，绘制其光谱，用 2851 cm^{-1}、1601 cm^{-1}、1028 cm^{-1}、907 cm^{-1} 处的吸收峰对仪器的波数进行校正。在 2000～400 cm^{-1} 区间允许相差 ±4 cm^{-1} 以内，在 4000～2000 cm^{-1} 区间允许相差 ±8 cm^{-1} 以内。

仪器分辨率要求在 3110～2850 cm^{-1} 范围以内应能清晰分辨出 7 个峰，2924 cm^{-1} 与 2851 cm^{-1} 吸收带的分辨深度不小于 18% 透光率，1601 cm^{-1} 与 1583 cm^{-1} 吸收带的分辨深度不小于 8% 透光率。仪器的分辨率，除另有规定外，应不低于 2 cm^{-1}。

（2）试样制备方法　用作鉴别时应按照药典委员会编订的《药品红外光谱集》第一卷（1995 年版）与第二卷（2000 年版）收载的各光谱图所规定的制备方法制备。

（3）有多晶现象的固体药品由于供测定的供试品晶型可能不同，导致绘制的光谱图与文献所收载的光谱图不一致。遇此情况时，应按该文献方法进行预处理后再绘制比较。

（4）由于各种型号仪器性能不同，试样制备时，研磨程度差异或吸水程度不同等原因，均会影响光谱形状。因此，进行光谱对比时，应考虑各种因素可能造成的影响。

六、色谱法

色谱法（又称层析法）根据其分离原理，分类如表 1-5 所示。

表1-5　根据分离原理色谱法的分类

色谱法	分离原理	固定相	流动相
吸附色谱	在吸附剂上吸附能力不同	氧化铝、硅胶、聚酰胺等有吸附活性的物质	溶剂或气体
分配色谱	在两相中分配系数的不同	被涂布或键合在固体载体，常用载体：硅胶、硅藻土、硅镁型吸附剂与纤维素粉	液体或气体
离子交换色谱	在离子交换色谱上交换能力的不同	阳离子交换树脂、阴离子交换树脂	水或含有机溶剂的缓冲液
凝胶色谱	被分离物质分子大小不同导致在填料上渗透程度不同	分子筛、葡聚糖凝胶、微孔聚合物、微孔硅胶或玻璃珠等	水或有机溶剂

色谱法又可根据分离方法分为：纸色谱法、薄层色谱法、柱色谱法、气相色谱法、高效液相色谱法等。所用溶剂应与供试品不起化学反应，纯度要求较高。分析时的温度，除气相色谱法或另有规定外，系指在室温操作。采用纸色谱法、薄层色谱法或柱色谱法分离有色物质时，可根据其色带进行区分；分离无色物质时，可在短波（254 nm）或长波（365 nm）紫外光等下检视，其中纸色谱或薄层色谱可喷以显色剂使之显色，或在薄层色谱中用加有荧光物质的薄层硅胶，采用荧光猝灭法检视。柱色谱法中气相色谱法和高效液相色谱法可于色谱柱出口处接各种检测器检测。柱色谱法还可分部收集流出液后用适宜方法测定。

（一）纸色谱法

纸色谱法以纸为载体，以纸上所含水分或其他物质为固定相，用展开剂展开的分配色谱。供试品经展开后，可用比移值（R_f）表示各组成成分的位置（比移值 = 原点中心至斑点中心的距离/原点中心至展开剂前沿的距离）。由于影响比移值的因素很多，因而一般采用在相同实验条件下与对照物质对比以确定其异同。作为药品的鉴别时，供试品在色谱中所现主斑点的位置与颜色（或荧光），应与对照品相同。作为药品的纯度检查时，可取一定量的供试品，经展开后，检视其所显杂质斑点的个数或呈色（或荧光）的强度。作为药品的含量测定时，将主色谱斑点剪下洗脱后，再用适宜的方法测定。

1. 仪器与材料

（1）展开室　通常为圆形或长方形玻璃缸，缸上具有磨口玻璃盖，应能密闭。用于下行法时，盖上有孔，可插入分液漏斗，用以加入展开剂。在近顶端有一用支架架起的玻璃槽作为展开剂的容器，槽内有一玻棒，用以压住色谱滤纸；槽的两侧各支一玻棒，用以支持色谱滤纸使其自然下垂，避免展开剂沿滤纸与溶剂槽之间发生虹吸现象。用于上行法时，在盖上的孔中加塞，塞中插入玻璃悬钩，以便将点样后的色谱滤纸挂在钩上；并除去溶剂槽和支架。

（2）点样器　常用微量注射器或定量毛细管，应能使点样位置正确、集中。

（3）滤纸　质地均匀平整，具有一定机械强度，不含影响展开效果的杂质；也不应与所用显色剂起作用，以致影响分离和鉴别效果，必要时可进行处理后再用。用于下行法时，取色谱滤纸按纤维长丝方向切成适当大小的纸条，离纸条上端适当的距离（使色谱纸上端能足够浸入溶剂槽内的展开剂中，并使点样基线能在溶剂槽侧的玻璃支持棒下数厘米处）用铅笔划一点样基线，必要时，可在色谱滤纸下端切成锯齿形便于展开剂滴下。用于上行法时，色谱滤纸长约25 cm，宽度则按需要而定，必要时可将色谱滤纸卷成筒形；点样基线距底边约2.5 cm。

2. 操作方法

（1）下行法　将供试品溶解于适当的溶剂中制成一定浓度的溶液。用微量吸管或微量注射器吸取溶液，点于点样基线上，溶液宜分次点加，每次点加后，待其自然干燥、低温烘干或经温热气流吹干。样点直径为2~4 mm，点间距离约为1.5~2.0 cm，样点通常应为圆形或带状。

将点样后的色谱滤纸上端放在溶剂槽内并用玻棒压住，使色谱纸通过槽侧玻璃支持棒自然下垂，点样基线在支持棒下数厘米处。展开前，展开缸内用各品种项下规定的溶剂蒸气饱和，一般可在展开缸底部放一装有规定溶剂的平皿或将浸有规定溶剂的滤纸条附着在展开缸内壁上，放置一定时间，待溶剂挥发使缸内充满饱和蒸气。然后添加展开剂，使其浸没溶剂槽内的滤纸，展开剂即经毛细作用沿滤纸移动进行展开，展开至规定的距离后，取出滤纸，标明展开剂前沿位置，待展开剂挥散后，按规定方法检出色谱斑点。

（2）上行法　点样方法同下行法。展开缸内加入展开剂适量，放置，待展开剂蒸气饱和后，再下降悬钩，使色谱滤纸浸入展开剂约0.5 cm，展开剂即经毛细作用沿色谱滤纸上升，除另有规定外，一般展开至约15 cm后，取出晾干，按规定方法检视。

展开可以向一个方向进行，即单向展开；也可进行双向展开，即先向一个方向展开，取出，待展开剂完全挥发后，将滤纸转动90°，再用原展开剂或另一种展开剂进行展开；亦可多次展开、连续展开或径向展开等。

（二）薄层色谱法

薄层色谱法，系将适宜的吸附剂或载体涂布于玻璃板、塑料或铝基片上，成一均匀薄层。经点样、展开后，与适宜的对照物按同法在同板上所得的色谱图对比，也可用薄层扫描仪进行扫描，用以进行药品的鉴别、杂质检查或含量测定的方法。

1. 仪器与材料

（1）玻板　除另有规定外，用10 cm×10 cm、10 cm×15 cm、20 cm×10 cm或20 cm×20 cm的规格，要求光滑、平整，洗净后不附水珠，晾干。

（2）吸附剂或载体　常用有：硅胶G、硅胶GF$_{254}$、硅胶H、硅胶HF$_{254}$，还有硅藻土、硅藻土G，氧化铝、氧化铝G、微晶纤维素、微晶纤维素F$_{254}$等。其颗粒大小一般要求直径为10~40 μm。薄层涂布，除另有规定外，一般可分无黏合剂和含黏合剂两种；前者系将吸附剂或载体用水适量调成糊状，均匀涂布于玻璃板上，后者系在吸附剂或载体中加入一定量的黏合剂，一般常用10%~15%煅石膏（CaSO$_4$·2H$_2$O在140℃加热4小时），混匀后加水适量使用，或用羧甲基纤维素钠水溶液（0.2%~0.5%）适量调成糊状，均匀涂布于玻璃板上。也有含一定改性剂如荧光剂或缓冲液等的薄层。

（3）涂布器　应能使吸附剂或载体在玻璃板上手工或自动涂成一层符合厚度要求

的均匀薄层。

（4）点样器　常用微量注射器或定量毛细管。

（5）展开室　可用适合薄层板大小的专用玻璃缸，底部平底或有双槽，盖子须密闭。

2. 操作方法

（1）薄层板制备　除另有规定外，将吸附剂 1 份和水 3 份在研钵中向一方向研磨混合，去除表面气泡后，倒入涂布器中，在玻板上平稳地移动涂布器进行涂布（厚度为 0.25 ~ 0.5 mm），取下涂好薄层的玻板，于室温下，置水平台上晾干，在反射光及透射光下检视，表面应均匀，平整，无麻点、无气泡、无破损及污染，于 110℃ 烘 30 分钟，冷却后立即使用或置干燥箱中备用。目前也有商品预制板。

（2）点样　用微量注射器或定量毛细管点样于薄层板上，一般为圆点（直径一般不大于 2 mm）或带状（长 3 ~ 8 mm），点样基线距底边 1.0 ~ 1.5 cm，点间距离可视斑点扩散情况以不影响检出为宜，点样时勿损伤薄层表面。

（3）展开　将点样的薄层板放入展开缸的展开剂中，浸入展开剂的深度为距原点 5 mm 为宜，密闭，待展开至规定距离，除另有规定外，一般为 8 ~ 15 cm，取出薄层板，晾干，按规定检测。

展开缸需预先用展开剂预平衡，在缸中加入适量的展开剂，在壁上贴一条与缸一样高、宽的滤纸条，一端浸入展开剂中，盖严。

3. 薄层扫描法　系指用一定波长的光照射在薄层板上，对薄层色谱中有吸收紫外光或可见光的斑点，或经激发后能发射出荧光的斑点进行扫描，将扫描得到的图谱及积分数据用于药品的鉴别、杂质检查或含量测定。

薄层扫描方法可根据各种薄层扫描仪结构特点及使用说明，结合具体情况，选择反射方式，采用吸收法或荧光法，双波长或单波长扫描。测定方法有内标法及外标法。由于影响薄层扫描结果的因素很多，故薄层扫描定量测定应在保证供试品斑点的量在校正曲线的线性范围内的情况下，与对照品同板点样，展开，扫描，积分和计算。

用外标法测定时，若对照品各数据点在校正曲线上呈一通过原点的直线时，可用一点法校正，如不通过原点通常宜采用二点法校正，必要时用多点法校正。含量测定时，供试品溶液应交叉点于同一薄层板上，供试品点样不得少于 4 个，对照品每一浓度不得少于 2 个，薄层扫描定量用的对照品纯度应符合含量测定用对照品的要求。

（三）柱色谱法

1. 吸附柱色谱　色谱柱为内径均匀、下端缩口的硬质玻璃管，下端用棉花或玻璃纤维塞住，管内装入吸附剂。吸附剂颗粒应尽可能保持大小均匀（通常直径为 0.07 ~ 0.15 mm 的颗粒），应控制色谱柱的大小，吸附剂的品种和用量，以及洗脱时的流速，以保证良好的分离效果。

（1）吸附剂填装

①干法　将吸附剂一次加入色谱柱，振动管壁使其均匀下沉，然后沿管壁缓缓加入洗脱剂；或在色谱柱下端出口处连接活塞，加入适量的洗脱剂，旋开活塞使洗脱剂缓缓滴出，然后自管顶缓缓加入吸附剂，使其均匀地润湿下沉，在管内形成松紧适度

的吸附层。操作过程中应保持有充分的洗脱剂留在吸附剂的上面。

②湿法 将吸附剂与洗脱剂混合，搅拌除去空气泡，徐徐倾入色谱柱中，然后加入洗脱剂将附着管壁的吸附剂洗下，使色谱柱面平整。

（2）供试品加入 一般将供试品溶于开始洗脱时使用的洗脱剂中，再沿管壁缓缓加入，注意勿使吸附剂翻起。或将供试品溶于适当的溶剂中，与少量吸附剂混匀，使溶剂挥尽呈松散状，加在已制备好的色谱柱上面。如供试品在常用溶剂中不溶，可将供试品与适量的吸附剂在乳钵中研磨混匀后加入。

（3）洗脱 通常按洗脱剂洗脱能力大小递增交换洗脱剂的品种和比例，分部收集流出液，至流出液中所含成分显著减少或不再含有时，再改变洗脱剂的品种和比例。操作过程中应保持有充分的洗脱剂留在吸附剂的上面。

2. 分配柱色谱 方法和吸附柱色谱基本一致。装柱前，先将载体和固定液混合，然后分次移入色谱柱中并用带有平面的玻棒压紧；供试品可溶于固定液，混以少量载体，加在预制好的色谱柱上端。洗脱剂需先加固定液混合使之饱和，以避免洗脱过程中两相分配的改变。

（四）高效液相色谱法

高效液相色谱法是用高压输液泵将具有不同极性的单一溶剂或不同比例的混合溶剂、缓冲液等流动相泵入装有固定相的色谱柱，经进样阀注入供试品，由流动相带入柱内，在柱内各成分被分离后，依次进入检测器，色谱信号由记录仪或积分仪记录。

1. 仪器的一般要求 所用的仪器为高效液相色谱仪。常用色谱柱填充剂有硅胶和化学键合硅胶，后者以十八烷基硅烷键合硅胶最为常用，辛烷基键合硅胶次之，氰基或氨基键合硅胶也有使用。离子交换填充剂用于离子交换色谱；凝胶或玻璃微球等填充剂用于分子排阻色谱；手性键合相填充剂用于对应异构体的拆分分析等。对于十八烷基硅烷键合硅胶为固定相的反相色谱系统，流动相中有机溶剂的比例通常应不低于5%，pH 范围宜控制在 2~8 范围内。

检测器为紫外吸收检测器或其他检测器，在用紫外吸收检测器时，所用流动相应符合紫外分光光度法项下对溶剂的要求。

正文中各品种项下规定的条件除固定相种类、流动相组分、检测器类型不得任意改变外，其余如色谱柱内径、长度、固定相牌号、载体粒度、流动相流速、混合流动相各组分的比例、柱温、进样量、检测器的灵敏度等，均可适当改变，选用适当具体条件以达到系统适用性试验的要求。一般色谱图约于 20 分钟内记录完毕。

2. 系统适用性试验 适用性试验，即用规定对照品对仪器进行试验和调整，应达到规定要求；或规定分析状态下色谱柱最小理论板数、分离度、重复性和拖尾因子。

（1）色谱柱理论板数（n） 在选定条件下，注入供试品溶液或内标物质溶液，记录色谱图，量出供试品主成分或内标物质峰的保留时间 t_R、半峰宽度（$W_{h/2}$），按 $n = 5.54 \, (t_R/W_{h/2})^2$ 计算色谱柱理论板数。如果测得理论板数低于规定的最小理论板数，应改变色谱柱的某些条件，如柱长、载体性能、色谱柱充填的优劣等，使理论板数达到要求。

（2）分离度 定量分析时，为便于准确测量，要求定量峰与其他峰或内标峰之间有较好的分离度。分离度一般应大于1.5。分离度（R）的计算公式为：

$$R = 2\ (t_{R_2} - t_{R_1})\ /\ (W_1 + W_2) \tag{1-3}$$

式中，t_{R_2}—相邻两峰中后一峰保留时间；

t_{R_1}—相邻两峰中前一峰保留时间；

W_1 及 W_2—相邻两峰的峰宽。

（3）重复性　取对照溶液，连续进样5次，其峰面积测量值的相对标准偏差一般应不大于2.0%。也可按校正因子测定，配制相当于80%、100%和120%的对照品溶液，加入规定量的内标溶液，配成3种不同浓度的溶液，分别进样3次，计算平均校正因子，其相对标准偏差也应不大于2.0%。

（4）拖尾因子　为保证测量精度，特别当采用峰高法测量时，应检查待测峰的拖尾因子（T）是否符合规定，或不同浓度进样的校正因子误差是否符合要求。T 一般应在 0.95～1.05 之间，计算公式为：

$$T = W_{0.05h}\ /\ (2d_1) \tag{1-4}$$

式中，$W_{0.05h}$—0.05 峰高处的峰宽；

d_1—峰顶点至峰前沿之间的距离。

3. 定量法　定量测定时，可根据供试品具体情况采用峰面积法或峰高法。测定杂质含量时，须采用峰面积法。

（1）内标法加校正因子测定供试品中某个杂质或主成分含量　精密称（量）取对照品和内标物质，分别配成溶液，精密量取各溶液，配成校正因子测定用的对照溶液。取一定量注入仪器，记录色谱图。测量对照品和内标物质的峰面积或峰高，按下式计算校正因子：

$$校正因子\ (f)\ = (A_S/c_S)\ /\ (A_R/c_R) \tag{1-5}$$

式中，A_S—内标物质的峰面积或峰高；

A_R—对照品的峰面积或峰高；

c_S—内标物质的浓度；

c_R—对照品的浓度。

再取各品种项下含有内标物质的供试品溶液，注入仪器，记录色谱图，测量供试品中待测成分（或其杂质）和内标物质的峰面积或峰高，按下式计算含量：

$$含量\ (c_X)\ = f \cdot A_X/\ (A_S/\ c_S) \tag{1-6}$$

式中，A_x—供试品（或其杂质）峰面积或峰高；

c_x—供试品（或其杂质）的浓度；

f、A_S 和 c_S 的意义同上。

当配制校正因子测定用的对照溶液和含有内标物质的供试品溶液使用同一份内标物质溶液时，则配制的内标物质溶液不必精密称（量）取。

（2）外标法测定供试品中某个杂质或主成分含量　按各品种项下的规定，精密称（量）取对照品和供试品，配制成溶液，分别精密取一定量，注入仪器，记录色谱图，测量对照品和供试品待测成分的峰面积（或峰高），按下式计算含量：

$$含量\ (c_X)\ = c_R \cdot\ (A_X/\ A_R)$$

式中各符号意义同上。

（3）加校正因子的主成分自身对照法　测定杂质含量时，可采用加校正因子的主成分自身对照法。在建立方法时，按各品种项下规定，精密称（量）取杂质对照品和待测成分对照品各适量，配制测定杂质校正因子的溶液，进样，记录色谱图，按上述（1）法计算杂质的校正因子。此校正因子可直接载入各品种正文中，用于校正杂质的实测峰面积。

测定杂质含量时，按各品种项下规定的杂质限度，将供试品溶液稀释成与杂质限度相当的溶液作为对照溶液，进样，调节仪器灵敏度（以噪声水平可接受为限）或进样量（以柱子不过载为限），使对照溶液的主成分色谱峰高约达满量程的 10%～25% 或其峰面积能准确积分（面积约为通常条件下满量程峰积分值的 10%）。然后，取供试品溶液和对照品溶液适量，分别进样，供试品溶液的记录时间除另有规定外，应为主成分保留时间若干倍，测量供试品溶液色谱图上各杂质的峰面积。分别乘以相应的校正因子后与对照溶液主成分的峰面积比较，依法计算各杂质含量。

（4）不加校正因子的主成分自身对照法　当没有杂质对照品时，可采用不加校正因子的主成分自身对照法。同上述（3）法配制对照溶液并调节仪器灵敏度后，取供试品溶液和对照溶液适量，分别进样，前者的记录时间除另有规定外，应为主成分保留时间的若干倍，测量供试品溶液色谱图上各杂质的峰面积并与对照溶液主成分的峰面积比较，计算杂质含量。

供试品所含的部分杂质未与溶剂峰完全分离，则按规定先记录供试品溶液的色谱图 I 再记录等体积纯溶剂的色谱图 II。色谱图 I 上杂质峰的总面积（包括溶剂峰），减去色谱图 II 上的溶剂峰面积，即为总杂质峰的校正面积。然后依法计算。

（5）面积归一化法　由于峰面积归一化法测定误差大，因此，本法通常只能用于粗略考察供试品中的杂质含量。除另有规定外，一般不宜用于微量杂质的检查。方法是测量各杂质峰的面积和色谱图上除溶剂峰以外的总色谱峰面积，计算各峰面积占总峰面积的百分率，即得。

由于微量注射器不易精确控制进样量，当采用外标法测定供试品中某杂质或主成分含量时，以定量环进样为好。

（五）气相色谱法

气相色谱法的流动相为气体，称为载气；色谱柱分为填充柱和毛细管柱两种：填充柱内装吸附剂、高分子多孔小球或涂渍固定液的载体，毛细管柱内壁或载体经涂渍或交联固定液。注入进样口的供试品被加热气化，并被载气带入色谱柱，在柱内各成分被分离后，先后进入检测器，色谱信号用记录仪或数据处理器记录。

1. 对仪器的一般要求　气相色谱仪除另有规定外，载气为氮气；色谱柱为填充柱或毛细管柱，填充柱材质为不锈钢或玻璃，载体用直径为 0.25～0.18 mm、0.18～0.15 mm 或 0.15～0.125 mm 经酸洗并硅烷化处理的硅藻土或高分子多孔小球；常用玻璃或弹性石英毛细管柱内径为 0.20 mm 或 0.32 mm。进样口温度应高于柱温 30～50℃；进样量一般不超过数微升；柱径越细进样量应越少。检测器为氢火焰离子化检测器，检测温度一般高于柱温，并不得低于 100℃，以免水汽凝结，通常为 250～350℃。

一般色谱图约于 30 分钟内记录完毕。

2. 系统适用性试验 除检测器种类、固定液品种及特殊指定的色谱柱材料不得任意改变外，其余如色谱柱内径、长度、载体牌号、粒度、固定液涂布浓度、载气流速、柱温，进样量、检测器的灵敏度等，均可改变，以符合系统适用性试验的要求。

3. 测定法 同高效液相色谱法。气相色谱法手工进样量不易精确控制，特别应注意留针时间和室温的影响。

（六）液相 - 质谱联用技术

严格来说，液相 - 质谱联用技术属于液相色谱法一种，由于质谱检测器的高灵敏度，既可以定性，又可以定量的独特优势，近年来在药物及其代谢产物、天然产物化学成分分析，残留物分析、生物大分子和临床诊断等方面应用非常广泛。事实上，气质联用较液质联用技术发展更早，但是气质联用技术对样品的要求较高，只有易气化的样品方能进行分析，多数样品需要经过适当的预处理或衍生化，而液相色谱可分离极性的、离子化的，不易挥发和热不稳定的化合物，可满足更多化合物的分析要求，具有更为广阔的应用前景。

液质联用的样品或流动相必须用 0.22 μm 滤膜过滤，不允许使用含不挥发盐组分的流动相。常用的离子源包括电喷雾离子源（ESI），大气压化学电离源（APCI），ESI 适合于中高级性的化合物，流速在 0.001 ~ 1 ml/min 范围内，检测分子量范围可以扩大到 30000 左右。APCI 适合于中低极性的中低分子量化合物，适合于分析分子量低于 1000 的样品，流速在 0.2 ~ 2 ml/min 范围内，ESI 的检测范围远比 APCI 广泛。在建立液质联用方法时，需对仪器参数，如电离方式、电离电压、离子源温度、脱溶温度、锥孔电压、流速、扫描范围等进行优化设置。

液质联用技术往往不需要进行系统适用性实验，谱图可以给出检测样品的分子量及二级裂解规律，从而对样品进行定性分析，同时可以给出检测样品的总离子流图或选择离子色谱图，采用内标法、外标法、标准曲线法进行定量分析。

Section 4　Physical and Chemical Identification and Quality Analysis of Crude Drugs

Physical and chemical identification is to carry out qualitative and quantitative analyses of effective constituents in crude drugs (including their preparation) by means of physical and chemical methods. It is the method to identify whether crude drugs are genuine and superior.

1. Qualitative analysis of chemical constituents

It can be used for identifying which kinds of chemical constituents are contained in crude drugs by using some chemical reagents to produce special colour or sediment.

2. Microscopic chemical reaction of crude drugs

Microscopic, physical and chemical identification are combined in this method. Generally put the powder, hand section or a bit of leachate on a slide, drop the proper reagent on it to make a temporary slice, test the sediment, crystal, bubble, dissolving and color change under microscope in order to identify the composition of cell wall, characteristics of ergastic substances in cells and distribution of some constituents. Thus we can discriminate some crude drugs. At the moment we are only introducing some of the methods.

(1) Composition of cell walls

① Lignificated cell walls   Generally put a fresh plant section on a slide, add 1 – 2 drops of 40% hydrochloric acid, wait for 3 – 5 min until the material is soaked, and add 5% phloroglucinol alcoholic solution. Ultimately the cell walls containing lignin will turn red or purple red. Vessels, tracheids, fibers and stone cells show obvious colors due to their abundant lignin; The experiment also can ensure the existence of Casparian dots in the endodermis cell walls due to plentiful lignin in those dots.

② Corkificated and cornified cell walls   Generally take a hand section or powder on a slide, add Sudan Ⅲ test solution, after cover with a coverslip, test under microscope and the corkificated cell walls will show orange red, red or purple red.

(2) Ergastic substances in cells

①Starch grains   Take a bit of powder on a slide, mount with iodine solution and starch grains will show blue or purple red.

②Calcium oxalate crystals   Take a little bit of powder on a slide, test under microscope, mount with dilute oxalic acid, calcium oxalate crystals can't dissolve; add 1 – 2 drops of dilute hydrochloric acid along the verge of coverslip, the calcium oxalate crystals will dissolve without bubbles. When we mount with 30% sulphuric acid (V/V), test under microscope, the calcium oxalate crystals dissolves and calcium sulfate raphides educe for a moment.

③ Protein (aleurone grains)   The protein stored in plants cells is abiotic, stable, amorphous, crystalline or fixed – shape aleurone grains. Aleurone grains are the main form of protein in the plant cells. Generally take some fresh materials on a slide, add 95% ethanol to dissolve fat, and then add iodine – potassium iodide solution, aleurone grains turn to yellow or brown grain.

④ Latex, fatty oil and volatile oil   Generally take some fresh material on a slide, add some of Sudan III solution, heat, cover with a coverslip and test under microscope, latex in lactifer, fatty oil and volatile oil are dyed into red.

(3) Microscopic chemical locating reaction   Determine the locations of effective constituents in plant tissue by means of microscopic and chemical methods. Generally take a hand section of fresh dehydrated materials on a slide, mount with some reagent, and test the color reaction and location under microscope. Take Radix bupleuri as an example; mount the section with the part. a eq. mixture of dehydrated alcohol and concentrated sulfuric acid, test under microscope, the color of saikosides location shows flavo – green initially, converts into green then to blue after 5 – 10 min which persists for more than one hour and then turns to dark blue and disappears ultimately.

3. Microsublimation

Some crude drugs contain the chemical constituents with sublimable characteristics at a certain temperature; microsublimation utilizes this character to get some sublimate with a microsublimating installation; observe the property, color and chemical reaction in order to identify the crude drugs. For example, both of rhubarb and fleeceflower root contained anthraquinone with sublimation characteristics can produce yellow needle crystals at low temperature, yellow plumery like needle crystals at a little high temperature and yellow oil drops at a high temperature. The crystals are dissolved when lye is added and the solution shows red, and then shows yellow when acid solution is added again. Cantharidin sublimate is colorless column crystals, dissolved in barium hydroxide solution and creats needle crystals. Paeonol sublimate in peony root bark is colorless needle, column or plumatus like crystals, dissolved in the chloride ferric solution and the solution shows dark purple.

The following is the process of microsublimation methods. Put a piece of tinsel on 1 slate, take a tiny metal ring (about 0.8 cm high) on the tinsel and a thin layer of crude drug powder in the ring which is covered with a glass slide. Heat with an alcohol lamp for several minutes until the powder begins to get scorched, cool, so crystal sublimate coagulates on the slide. Reverse the slide, cover with a coverslip, observe the form of crystals with a microscope, then add some reagent, observe the reaction result. Determine the melting point with a microscopic melting point determinator if necessary.

4. Fluorimetric analysis

It is a simple method to identify crude drugs contained some kind of chemical constituents with the fluorescence characteristics under ultraviolet light or natural light. Generally take the cut crude drug, powder or their extract, irradiate under a fluoroscope in dark. For example, the cut crude drug of golden thread shows orange fluorescence, the rhubarb powder shows dark brown and water ext. of ash bark shows sapphire.

Some crude drugs though do not possess fluorescence characteristics, when acid, alkali or other chemical reagent reacts with them, their contained constituents can show fluorescence. For example, aloe's water ext. shows no fluorescence, but it shows flavo – green fluorescence as heated with borax due to contained aloetin. We can also carry out quantitative assay with a fluoreanalyzer according to fluorescent intensity of crude drugs. The lichen or fungus attached on the surface of crude drugs may also generate fluorescence. So we can check the transformation of crude drugs.

Further we can also identify the crude drugs with a fluorescence microscope, for example, the powder of domestic eaglewood shows marine blue to celadon, but the imported one shows green.

5. Spectrophotometry

Spectrophotometry is a kind of qualitative and quantitative analysis method for some kind of substance through measuring its absorbability at certain wavelength or certain wavelength scope.

Wavelength	Light zone	Measuring apparatus
200 – 400 nm	Ultraviolet light	UV spectrophotometer
400 – 760 nm	Visible light	Spectrophotometer or chromometer
2. 5 – 25 mm (wave number 4000 – 400 cm^{-1})	Infrared light	Infrared spectrophotometer Atomicabsorption spectrometer

When monochromatic light goes through the measured solution, the quantity absorbed by some substance is proportional to solution concentration and liquid thickness (length of optical path); their relationship is as the following formula:

$$A = \lg \ (1/T) \ = Ecl$$

A: absorbability; T: transmittancy; E: absorption coefficient ($E_{1\,cm}^{1\%}$), its physical sense is the absorbability value when the solution concentration is 1% (g/ml) and the solution thickness is 1 cm; c: the quality of measured substance in 100 ml solution (g, refers to dried or anhydrous substance); l: solution thickness (1 cm).

The absorption wavelength and absorption coefficient are kinds of physical constants of some substance. So if the absorption coefficient of some pure substance is known, we can prepare its test sample contained this pure constituent into solution in a similar condition and measure its absorbability. In this way we can get the content of the pure constituent in the test solution.

In the visible light zone, except for some substance, many have not optical absorption, but they may be measured absorbability if a coloring reagent is added and this method is named colorimetric analysis. Because many factors influence coloring and the instruments with impure monachromatic light are always used, we should measure the standard preparation and control article at the same time.

(1) Ultraviolet spectrophotometry

① Calibration and standardization of instruments   The instrument wavelength always alternates because mechanical part is usually influenced by change of temperature, so we should not only calibrate the instrument completely and periodically, but also rectify the measuring wavelength before using. The stronger spectral lines in a common mercury lamp are 237. 83 nm, 253. 65 nm, 275. 28 nm, 296. 73 nm, 313. 16 nm, 334. 15 nm, 365. 02 nm, 404. 66 nm, 435. 8 nm, 546. 07 nm and 576. 96 nm; in deuterium lamp are 486. 02 nm and 656. 10 nm spectral lines; holmium glass possesses sharp absorption peaks at wavelength 279. 4 nm, 287. 5 nm, 333. 7 nm, 360. 9 nm, 418. 5 nm, 460. 0 nm, 484. 5 nm, 532. 6 nm and 637. 5 nmm, which also could be used for calibrating wavelength; but should pay attention to the tiny difference of wavelength emitted by different light sources.

Checking of absorbability accuracy: Take about 60 mg of potassium dichromate which has dried until its weight is constant at 120℃, weigh precisely, dissolve into 1000 ml of 0.005mol/L sulphuric acid solution, determine and calculate its absorption coefficient at the defined wavelength; then compare with the defined absorption coefficient as the list below and the relative standard deviation should be less than 1%.

Wavelength (nm)	235 (mini)	257 (max)	313 (mini)	350 (mini)
Absorption coefficient ($E_{1\,cm}^{1\%}$)	124.5	144.0	48.62	106.6

The determination of stray light: Prepare their water solution according to the reagents and concentrations in the below table, put them into the quartz cell (1 cm), and determine the transmittancy at the defined wavelength as the listed below.

Reagent	Concentration (%, g/ml)	Wavelength (nm)	Transmittancy (%)
sodium iodide	1.00	220	<0.8
sodium nitrite	5.00	340	<0.8

②Requests for solvents We should examine whether a solvent has absorption at the wavelength used by a test sample before measuring the test sample, fill the 1 cm quartz cell with the solvent, and measure its absorbability with air as the blank (nothing is laid in the blank beam path). The absorbability of a solvent and absorption cell should be less than 0.40 in the scope of 220 – 240 nm, less than 0.20 in the scope of 241 – 250 nm, less than 0.10 in the scope of 251 – 300 nm and less than 0.05 above 300 nm.

③ Measuring methods In measuring, we should use the same batch of solvent prepared for a test solution as the blank solution, use 1 cm quartz absorption cell, and measure the absorbability of the test sample at several points within ±2 nm of the defined wavelength to examine whether its absorption wavelength is correct. Except for other rules, the absorption wavelength should be within the scope of ±2 nm of the defined wavelength for this substance. Otherwise we should think about the trueness and purity of the sample, precision of the instrument wavelength, and whether we measure the sample at the maximal absorption wavelength. Generally the reading error is little when absorbability is within 0.3 – 0.7. The width of slit wavestrip of instruments should be less than that of absorption band of a test sample; otherwise the measured absorbability will be lower. Here is a standard for choosing the slit width: decrease the slit width until the absorbability of a teat sample stops increasing; because the absorption cell and solution themself may also have absorption; the measured absorbability of the test sample should subtract the blank absorption, and then calculate its content.

The methods of assaying:

I. Comparison method with a control article Prepare a test sample and control article solution with the same solvent, the measured constituent content in the control article solution should be 100% ±10% of its marked content in the test sample. After measure the absorbability of the test sample and control article solution at the defined wavelength, calculate the measured constituent content in the test sample according to the formula below:

$$c_X = (A_X / A_R) \, c_R$$

In this formula, c_X: content of the test sample; A_X: absorbability of the test sample; c_R: concentration of the control article; A_R: absorbability of the control article.

II. Calculating with absorption coefficient　Prepare a test sample in the defined way and after measuring the absorbability of the contained constituent at the set wavelength, calculate its content by using the defined absorption coefficient. We should calibrate and examine the instrument when we use this method.

III. Calculation spectrophotometry　Be cautious to use this method. It can be used in many ways. If absorbability is measured at the wavelength where a absorption curve rises or descends sharply, the tiny change of wavelength will have a great influence on the measured results, so the measuring conditions of a control article and test sample should be almost the same. If we measure absorbability of a test sample without control article, such as vitamin A, we should calibrate and examine the instrument carefully.

(2) Colorimetry　A control article should be measured with a test sample at the same time when we use this method. The blank solution in colorimetry is to use the same volume solvent to take place of the control article. Then add corresponding reagents in the same quantity in turns and operating by the same method as to the test sample. Measure the absorbability of the control article and test sample at the set wavelength and calculate the test sample content according to the formula in comparison method [in (I)].

When the relationship between the absorbability and concentration don't show linearity, take several portions of the control article solution in gradient quantity, add solvent to the same volume, measure their absorbability after coloration, draw a standard curve with the absorbability and corresponding concentration and then calculate the content according to the test sample absorbability on the standard curve.

(3) Infrared spectrophotometry

① Instrument and calibration　Fourier transformation infrared spectrometer or dispersion infrared spectrophotometer is calibrated by polystyrene film (the thickness is about 0.05 nm), draw its spectrum and calibrate wave number according to the absorption peaks of polystyrene film at the 2851 cm^{-1}, 1601 cm^{-1}, 1028 cm^{-1}, 907 cm^{-1}. The permitted discrepancy is within ± 4 cm^{-1} in 2000 – 400 cm^{-1}, and ± 8 cm^{-1} in 4000 – 2000 cm^{-1}.

7 peaks must be discriminated clearly in 3110 – 2850 cm^{-1}, according to the instrument resolution requirement, difference in depth is not less than 18% of transmittancy at the absorption bands of 2924 cm^{-1} and 2851 cm^{-1}, and not less than 8% of transmittancy at 1601 cm^{-1} and 1583 cm^{-1}. Generally the resolution is not less than 2 cm^{-1}, except for other rules.

② Preparation methods　Prepare a test sample according to the methods in < Collection of medical infrared spectra > revised by the pharmacopeia committee, noted in the first volume

(1995 edition) and in the second volume (2000 edition).

③ The solid test samples with heteromorphism may give different crystal forms, which can make their spectrograms different. So we should measure spectra after pretreatment according to methods in literatures.

④ It will affect the spectra shape by different functions of various types of instruments and different grinding degrees and hydrating degrees of the prepared test sample. Therefore, we should consider all the influence factors when compare the spectra.

6. Stratography

Stratography (also called stratographic analysis) can be divided into the following types according to the separation principle.

Stratography	Separation principle	Stationary phase	Mobile phase
Chromatographic absorption	different adsorbabilities on adsorbens	substances with adsorbability like aluminium oxide, silica gel, polyamide, etc	solvent or gas
Chromatographic partition	different partition coefficients in two phases	coated or linked with Solid carrier like silica gel, kieselguhr, Si – Mg adsorbent and celluflour	liquid or gas
Chromatography of ions	different exchange capacity in chromatography of ions	cation and anion exchange resins	water or buffer contained organic solvent
Chromatograph of gel permeation	different permeation degree on the stuffing due to the different molecule size of an isolated substance	molecular sieve, polydextran gel, microporous polymer, micropore silica gel, glass pearls, etc	water ororganic solvent

Stratography can be divided into paper chromatography, thin layer chromatography, column chromatography, gas chromatography, and high performance liquid chromatography according to separation methods. The used solvent with high purity doesn't react with a test sample normally, except for in the special case or GC, usually at room temperature. The colorful sample can be separated with PC, TLC or CC according to color bars. When colorless substance is separated, it can be examined under an ultraviolet light at short wave (254 nm) or long wave (365 nm) and a chromogenic agent can be used in PC or TLC, or use fluorescent materials in their stationary phase for TLC and detect it by fluorescence quenching. As for GC and HPLC, we can set up several detectors at their chromatographic column outlet. We may measure the collected effluent portions with proper methods in column chromatography.

(1) Paper chromatography   Paper chromatography belongs to partition chromatography, in which, paper is used as a carrier, and water or other substances on the paper as its stationary phase, and develop with developing solvent. After developing, the positions of each moity

can be indicated by flow rate (R_f = the distance between the original point center and spot center/the distance between the original point center and solvent front) . Because many factors can influence R_f value, usually compared with that of a control article in same condition, R_f value of a test sample is identified. As an identification method of drugs, the position and color of the main spots of a test drug sample should be identical to those of a control article. As a purity identification method, a test sample weighed exactly is developed and then is examined the numbers and coloration (or fluorescence) intensity of impurity spots. As a content assay method, cut out and elute the spots, then examine with proper methods.

① Instruments and materials

I. Developing chamber It is usually a round or rectangle glass trough covered with a ground glass tightly. In descending method, there is bore on the cover to insert a tap funnel for adding developing solvent. The container of developing solvent is made of glass trough with a bracket near to top, in which there is a glassy stick to fix a piece of filter paper, on two sides of which two glassy sticks support the filter paper to droop naturally in order not to generate siphonage between the filter paper and developer trough. Using the champer in ascending method, bung the bore of cover and remove the solvent trough and bracket, insert a glass hook in the bung in order to hang the spotting filter paper.

II. Sample applicator Microsyringe or quantitative capillary is usually used to make the right position and concentration of spotting.

III. Filter paper It should be flat and be of uniform texture, with proper mechanical strength, without impurity, not to react with chromogenic agents to influence separating effects and to be processed further if necessary. In descending method, cut filter paper into slips in proper size along the fiber filement, draw a spotting base line away proper distance from the top of slip by a pencil (in order to immerse the slip top into the solvent and make the line several centimeters below the supporting glass stick in the solvent trough); cut the slip bottom into serration to make the developing solvent drop easily if necessary. In ascending method, the length of filter paper is about 25 cm, the width is decided by experimental demands; roll into cylinder form if necessary; the spotting base line is about 2.5 cm away from bottom.

② Operating methods

I. Descending method Dissolve a test sample with proper solvent to make the sample solution at certain concentration. Imbibe the solution with a micropipette or microsyringe, apply samples in fractionation on baseline, airdry, torrefy at low temperature or blow each droping fraction by heated air. The spot diameter is $2-4$ cm and the distance in two spots is $1.5-2.0$ cm; the spot should be round or barred.

Put the chromatographic filter paper in the solvent trough and its top fixed with glass sticks on 2 sides to make the paper droped naturally, the baseline is several centimeters below the supporting stick. Saturate the solvent trough with defined solvent before developing and generally put in a flat plate full of the solvent on bottom or attach paper strips soaked by the solvent on the champer wall. Add the developer to immerse the paper until the container is full of the saturated vapor, develop (capillary action) to the set distance, take out the paper, sign the position of the solvent front, evaporate the developer and examine the spots according to some methods.

Ⅱ. Ascending method   The spotting methods are the same as in the descending method. Put proper developer into the container, drop out a hook until the developer vapor is saturated, make the slip immersed into the developer 0.5 cm, take out the slip and air dry until the developer goes along paper 15 cm by capillary action and then examine according to some methods.

Developing towards one direction is called one – dimensional development; two – dimensional development is to develop firstly in one direction, then take out and evaporate the solvent, turn the paper for 90° and develop with the primary or another developer; there are also multiple development, continuous development and radial development.

(2) Thin layer chromatography   Thin layer chromatography is to coat some special absorbent or carrier on glass plates, plastic or aluminium chips to form a uniform thin layer. After spotting and developing the plate, compare their chromatogram with a control artical on the same plate, or scan with a thin – layer chromatogram scanner to carry out identification, impurity test or assaying.

① Instruments and materials

Ⅰ. Glass plate   Except for special rules, 10 cm × 10 cm, 10 cm × 15 cm, 20 cm × 10 cm or 20 cm × 20 cm types can be used; they should be clean, slick, flat and without water globules.

Ⅱ. Adsorbents and carriers   The common used types are Silica gel G, silica gel GF_{254}, silica gel H, silica gel HF_{254}, and also kieselguhr, kieselguhr G, alumina, alumina G, cellulose, cellulose F_{254}, etc, with 10 – 40 μm of particle diameter. Lamellar spreading can be divided into two types: without or with adhesive; the former is to make the adsorbent or carrier pasty with water, coat on the plate uniformly; the later is to add adhesive which is usually 10% – 15% dried gypsum (heat $CaSO_4 \cdot 2H_2O$ at 140℃ for 4 hours), mix with proper water, or make it to be pasty with sodium carboxymethycellulose (0.2% – 0.5%), coated on the plate. We can also add modifier like fluorescent agent or buffer.

Ⅲ. Spreader   It needs to coat a thin layer with uniform thickness of a kind of adsorbent or carrier on the glass plate manually or automatically.

Ⅳ. Sample applicator   It usually is a microinjector or quantitative capillary.

Ⅴ. Developing chamber   It is a special glass trough in proper size, with flat bottom or two grooves and a tightly – closed cover.

② Operating methods

Ⅰ. Preparation of thin layer plate   Grind the adsorbent and water (1:3) towards the same direction in a mortar, remove the bubbles on surface, pour into a spreader, coat on glass plate with the spreader steadily (thickness is 0.25 – 0.5 mm), dry the prepared plate in the open – air at room temperature on a level table, examine with reflected and transmitted light to make sure that it is flat, uniform and without pocks, bubbles, breakage and contamination, roast for 30 min at 110℃ and use it after cooled or reserved. Now there are commercial precoated plates.

Ⅱ. Spotting Apply the samples on plate with 1microsyringe or quantitative capillary. The application spots are usually round (diameter is less than 2 mm) or girdle – shaped (length is 3 – 8 mm), the spots are 1.0 – 1.5 cm apart from the bottom edge and the distance between two spots is adapt to develop. Spotting can not break the adsorbent on plate.

Ⅲ. Developing Immerse the plate into developer of chromatographic tank 5 mm away from the baseline, close tightly with cover, develop to the rated distance (is usually 8 – 15 cm), take out the plate, dry in the open – air and examine according to some methods.

The chromatographic tank should be saturated with the developer firstly. Add proper developer; paste a piece of filter paper with the same length and width as those of the tank on the wall with one end immersed in the developer and then cover tightly.

③ TLC scanning method Irradiate thin layer plate with light at some wavelength to scan the spots which can generate ultraviolet or visible light or fluorescence after excited. The spectrum or integral data obtained from scanning can be used for identifying, impurity test or assay of drugs.

Scanning methods (reflection mode, absorption or fluorometric method, double or single wavelength scanning) can be applied according to scanner characteristics and operating instruction. The assay methods include internal and external standard methods. Due to many influencing factors on scanning result, we should ensure that the quantity of a test sample spot is in the linear range of calibration trace, then apply the test sample with a control article on the same plate, develop, scan, integrate and calculate.

As to external reference method, if the calibration trace formed by a control article data crosses the original point, we can calibrate according to one – point method; if not, do according to two – point method, to multipoint method if necessary. As to assaying, a test sample solution should be applied interlacedly with a control article on the same plate, the spotting points of the test sample should not be less than 4, that of the control article with the same concentration must not be less than 2 and the purity of the control article in TLC scanning should meet the assaying request.

(3) Column chromatography

① Adsorption column chromatography The column is a rigid glass tube with uniform inside diameter and a retracting base, the base is stopped up by cotton or glass fiber, put a kind of adsorbent into the tube, whose particle diameter should be uniform (usually is 0.07 – 0.15 mm). Column size, type, quantity of the adsorbent and elution flow rate should be controlled in order to get good separating effect.

Ⅰ. Loading adsorbent

Dry process：

Load all the adsorbent one time, shake well to make it uniformly distributed, add eluant gradually along the tube wall; or link a stopcock on the outlet at base, add proper eluent, open the stopcork to make the eluent drop gradually and add the adsorbent from tube top to make it sink gradually to form moderate tightness adsorption layer. In the process we should keep eluent above the adsorbent.

Wet process：

Mix the adsorbent and eluent together, stir to remove bubbles, pour it into the column, and then add eluent to wash down the adsorbent attached on the tube wall and make the adsorbent surface flat.

Ⅱ. Adding a test sample　Dissolve a test sample in primary used eluent, and then load it into the tube along the wall avoiding for making the adsorbent upflated. Or dissolve a test sample with proper solvent, mix with a bit of adsorbent, then evaporate the solvent to make the mixture loose, load it into the prepared chromato bar. If a test sample doesn't dissolve in common solvent, we can grind it with some adsorbent together, and then load it into.

Ⅲ. Elution　Usually change the type and ratio of eluent according to the increasing of eluting power, collect the effluent fractions until the constituent in effluent decreases significantly or vanishes, then alter the type and ratio of eluent. In the process we should keep eluent above the adsorbent.

② Partition column chromatography　The methods are almost the same as adsorption column chromatography. Mix the carrier and stationary liquid together, put them into column in fractionation, press out by a glass stick with a flat end; or dissolve a test sample in a little of stationary liquid, add a small amount of carrier, load it into the prepared chromato bar. Saturate the eluent with stationary liquid to avoid for change of two – phase partition in elution process.

（4）High performance liquid chromatography　High performance liquid chromatography is to pump single solvent with different polarities or mixed solvent（buffer）with different ratios into a chromatographic column loaded stationary phase with a high pressure infusion pump, inject test sample through sampling valve, bring the sample into column by mobile phase, in which each component is separated and then flow into detector one by one, in which the color spectrum signals produced by these constituents are recorded by a recorder or integrator.

①General request for instruments　In this method, high performance liquid chromatograph is applied. The loading agents of common column are silica gel and chemical bonded silica gel; the latter are usually octadecyl and octyl silane and cyano or amino chemical bonded silica gel. Ion loading agent is applied in ion exchange chromatography; gel and glass microballoons are applied in size exclusion chromatography; charity bonded phase is used in the separation and analysis of enantiomers. For octadecyl and octyl silane chemical bonded silica gel column, the ratio of organic solvent in mobile phase should not be less than 5% and the pH value should be controlled within 2 – 8.

Ultraviolet absorption detector is usually applied. As to the ultraviolet absorption detector, the mobile phase should meet the request to ultraviolet spectrophotometry.

According to the rules in books, the types of stationary phase, detectors and constituents of mobile phase cannot be changed at will; however, other chromatographic conditions such as the inside diameter of chromato bar, length, brand of stationary phase, particle size of carrier, flow rate of mobile phase, the ratio of mixed mobile phase, column temperature, sample size and sensitivity of detector may be changed to meet the request of system suitability. Generally 1 chromatogram should be finished record within 20 min.

② System suitability test   Suitability test is to examine and adjust the instruments with the defined control article to make them meet requirement; or analyse minimum of the theoretical plate number, resolving power, reproducibility and tailing factor in the rated conditions.

Ⅰ. Theoretical plate number (n)   In some conditions, inject a test sample solution or internal standard substance solution, record its chromatogram, get the retention time (t_R) and half – peak width ($W_{h/2}$) of the peaks of principal constituents in the test sample or internal standard, calculate the minimum of theoretical plate number according to the formula of $n = 5.54 \ (t_R/W_{h/2})^2$. If the minimum of theoretical plate number we measured is less than the rated value, some conditions such as the column length, carrier performance and filling of chromatographic column should be changed to meet the rated requirements.

Ⅱ. Resolving power   As to quantitative analysis, it requires good resolving power between the sample peak and other peaks (including the internal standard peak) for an accurate calculation. The resolution usually should be more than 1.5. The formula for resolution (R) is:

$$R = 2 \ (t_{R_2} - t_{R_1}) \ / \ (W_1 + W_2)$$

In this formula, t_{R_2}: the retention time of the posterior one in two borders upon peaks; t_{R_1}: the retention time of the anterior peak; W_1, W_2: the peak width of the two peaks.

Ⅲ. Repeatability   Take a control article solution, inject for 5 times continuously into HPLC, the relative standard deviation of their peak area should not be more than 2.0%. The correction factor also can be used to value repeatability, in which prepare 80%, 100% and 120% of control article solution, add the rated quantity of an internal standard solution to prepare 3 kinds of solution in different concentrations, inject 3 times respectively, calculate the average correction factor, and their relative standard deviation should not be more than 2.0%.

Ⅳ. Tailing factor   To ensure the measuring precision, especially when calculate by the method of peak height, examine whether the tailing factor (T) or correction factor error produced by different injection concentrations meet requirement. Generally T should be in 0.95 – 1.05, and its calculation formula is:

$$T = W_{0.05h} / \ (2d_1)$$

In the formula, $W_{0.05h}$: the peak width at peak height of 0.05; d_1: the distance between the peak top to peak front edge.

③ Quantitative method   As to quantitative assay, we can use method of peak area or peak height according to different samples. As to the impurity content, we should apply the former.

I. Content assaying of main constituent or impurity with the correction factor and method of internal standard   Weigh some control article and internal standard substance precisely, dissolve them into some solvent, take accurately each solution and make contrast solutions for correction factor determination. Inject some into HPLC and record the chromatogram, measure the peak area or height of the control article and internal standard substance and calculate the correction factor according to the following formula:

$$\text{Correction factor } (f) = (A_S/c_S) / (A_R/c_R)$$

In this formula, A_S: the peak area or height of an internal standard substance; A_R: the peak area or height of a control article; c_S: the concentration of the internal standard substance; c_R: the concentration of the control article.

Take a sample solution contained the rated internal standard substance, inject into HPLC and record its chromatogram, calculate the peak area or height of the internal standard substance and test constituent (or its impurity) in the sample, and then calculate its concentration according to the following formula:

$$\text{Content } (c_X) = f \cdot A_X / (A_S/ c_S)$$

In this formula, A_X: the peak area or height of a tested constituent (or its impurity); c_X: the concentration of the tested constituent (or its impurity); f, A_S and c_S have the same meanings as the above.

If we apply the same internal standard substance in the two formul as above, the internal standard substance need not to be measured precisely.

II. Content assaying of the main constituent or some impurity in a test sample by the method of external standard   Weigh a control article and test sample precisely according to prescription, dissolve them into some solvent, take out some of them precisely, inject into HPLC, record the chromatogram, calculate the peak area (or height) of the control article and main constituent in the test sample and calculate the content according to the following formula:

$$c_X = c_R \cdot (A_X / A_R)$$

All the symbols show the ditto meanings.

III. Assaying of own control with the correction factor of a principal constituent   This method can be used for impurity assay. To establish the method, weigh a control article of some kind of impurity and test constituent precisely, dissolve them into some solvent according to the method for measuring the impurity correction factor, inject into HPLC, record the chromatogram, calculate this kind of impurity correction factor according to the method (I) as above. The correction factor can be used to correct the real peak area of impurity.

As to the assaying of impurity content, dilute a test sample solution to the concentration corresponding to the defined impurity limit as a contrast solution, inject into HPLC, adjust sensitivity of the instrument (limit to the accepted noise level) or quantity of the injected sample （limit to no overloading to column）to make peak height of the major constituent in the contrast solution to 10% − 25% of total peak height or make its peak area can be integrated precisely （usually about 10% of the full range integral）. Then take some of the test sample and control article solution, inject respectively, the record time of the test sample usually should be several times of that of the major constituent, calculate the peak area of each impurity in the sample solution according to the chromatogram, multiply the corresponding correction factors, compare with peak area of major constituent in the contrast solution and calculate each impurity content according to the rated formula.

Ⅳ. Assaying of own control without correction factor of the principal constituent   We use this method when an impurity control article is absent. Prepare the contrast solution as method （Ⅲ）and adjust sensitivity of instrument, take some of the test sample and contrast solution, inject into HPLC respectively, the record time of the test sample should be several times of that of the major constituent, measure the impurity peaks area of the test sample in its chromatogram and compare with that of the major constituent in the contrast solution, and then calculate each impurity content.

If some impurity peaks in a test sample are not separated from solvent peak completely, firstly record the chromatogram I of the test sample solution and then chromatogram II of pure solvent with the same volume. All area（including the solvent peaks）of total impurity peaks in chromatogram I is subtracted by the solvent peaks area in chromatogram II, so get calibrating area of total impurity peaks, and then calculate with the rated methods.

Ⅴ. Area normalization method   This method is only used for calculating impurity content in a test sample roughly and not suitable to check microscale impurity. In this method, calculate the peak area of each impurity and total peaks area（not including solvent peak）to get the percentage of each impurity peak in total peaks.

When calculate the content of some impurities or major constituent in a test sample by external reference method, a ration ring must be used because a microsyringe can't control the sample size precisely.

（5）Gas chromatography   The mobile phase in this method is gas called carrier gas; chromatographic column can be divided into packed column and capillary column. The packed column is loaded with some adsorbent, porous polymer beads or carrier coated with stationary liquid; the capillary column wall or carrier are coated or cross − linked with stationary liquid. The injected test sample is gasified, and carried into column by carrier gas; when constituents are separated and flow into the detector, recorder or data processor records their chromatographic signals.

① General request to instrument   Its carrier gas is usually Nitrogen gas; its column is packed or capillary column, the packed materials are stainless steel or glass, the carrier is acid pickled and processed kieselguhr or porous polymer beads with silylation, with diameter of 0. 25 − 0. 18 mm, 0. 18 − 0. 15 mm or 0. 15 − 0. 125 mm; the inside diameter of common glass or quartz capillary column is 0. 22 mm or 0. 32 mm. The injecting opening temperature should be 30 – 50℃ higher than column temperature; Sample size is usually less than several microliters, the thinner column is, and the smaller sample size is. The detector is usually a flame ionization detector, detecting temperature should be higher than column temperature but not lower than 100℃ so that water vapor cannot condense, the common temperature is 250 – 350℃.

Generally the chromatogram should be recorded within 30 min.

② System suitability test   Detector type, stationary liquid and column materials should not be changed as will, the other parameters, like the inside diameter, length of column, carrier brand, particle size, spreading concentration of stationary liquid, flow rate of carrier gas, column temperature, sample size and detector sensitivity may change to meet the requests of system suitability test.

③ Assay   It is the same as that in HPLC. Sample size of GC cannot be controlled precisely, pay more attention to the influences of needle – remaining time and room temperature.

(6) HPLC – MS Analysis   Strictly speaking, HPLC – MS belong to the category of LC method. Just due to the high sensitivity and the unique advantage of MS detection that could accomplish quantitation and qualification simultaneously, HPLC – MS was widely used in the analysis of metabolites, natural products, trace compounds, bio – macromolecule and clinic diagnosis in recent years. In fact, GC – MS was earlier applied and developed than HPLC – MS. However, the sample for GC – MS need more strictly screening, only the sample easily to be pneumatolytic could be analyzed so that many samples need further pretreatment or derivatization, Which limits its application. The HPLC could separate the compounds which are polar, ionized, less volatile and heat – labile, meeting the most analysis requirement of samples and owning more expansive application prospect.

The sample or the mobile phase should be filtered with 0. 22 μm membrane before analysis. Non – volatile salt was forbidden in the mobile phase. The common ion source includes ESI and APCI. ESI is fit for the ionizing of compounds with middle or high polarity, the flow is often within 0. 001 – 1 ml/min, the detection molecular mass could be around 30 000. APCI is fit for the ionizing of compounds with middle or low polarity, the flow is often within 0. 2 – 2 ml/min, the detection molecular mass is less than 1 000. The detection field of ESI was much wider than APCI. During the establishment of HPLC – MS method, some parameters like ionization methods, ionization voltage, ion source temperature, desolventizing temperature, taper hole voltage, flow and scanned range should be optimized.

Usually, System suitability test is not necessary in HPLC – MS method. The spectrum could supply the molecular weight and the secondary decomposition fragment, which could help for the qualifications of compounds, and also supply the Total Ion Chromatography and Select ion chromatograms, which could help for the quantitation of compounds using the method of internal standard method, external standard method or standard curve method.

第五节 生药的 DNA 分子鉴定

随着分子生物学技术的发展，诞生了多种类型的分子标记鉴别技术，生药分子鉴定是在生物 DNA 分子多态性的基础上建立起来的，运用 DNA 分子标记技术对生药进行真伪优劣的鉴定，以确定其基源，评价其质量的一种较新的生药鉴定方法。

一、限制性片段长度多态性（Restriction Fragment Length Polymorphism, RFLP）标记技术

RFLP 标记是发展最早的 DNA 标记技术，是一项通过显示限制性酶切片段的大小检测不同遗传位点等位变异（多态性）的一种技术。

对于不同种群或居群的生物个体而言，它们的 DNA 序列存在多态性差别，产生的原因主要源自两种突变方式：一是限制性内切酶识别位点上发生单个碱基突变，使原有酶切位点消失或产生新的位点；二是由于片段缺失或插入导致酶切片段的长度发生改变。当利用同一种限制性内切酶切割不同物种或不同居群的 DNA 序列时，由于目标 DNA 既有同源性又有变异，因而酶切片段长度就有差异，产生不同长度大小、不同数量的限制性酶切片段。

目前 RFLP 标记技术常与 PCR 技术联合使用，即首先采用 PCR 技术，扩增得到包括某一个或数个多态性的限制性内切酶识别序列的等位特异性 DNA 序列片段，扩增产物再经该内切酶切割后电泳分离。根据获得的限制性片段长度多态性分布，判断不同等位基因的特异性，达到鉴定的目的。PCR – RFLP 标记可对微量的 DNA 样品进行分析，且无需测序，仪器限制较少，但需要事先设计并合成可扩增目的序列的引物。

二、随机扩增 DNA 多态性（random amplified polymorphic DNA, RAPD）标记技术

RAPD 标记技术是基于 PCR 技术的一种可对整个基因组进行多态性分析的遗传标记技术。该技术常使用随机引物进行 PCR，对于不同模板的 DNA，用同一引物进行扩增既可得到相同电泳谱带（高同源模板基因组），也可能会得到不同的电泳谱带，这样就可通过同种引物扩增条带的多态性反映出模板 DNA 的多态性。

RAPD 实验流程和 PCR 相似，包括样品 DNA 的提取及其纯度和浓度检测、PCR 扩增、产物电泳检测、实验数据分析等步骤。但一般使用较低的退火温度如 36°C，以保证引物与模板的稳定结合，同时允许适当的错误配对，以扩大引物在基因组 DNA 中的配对随机性，提高 RAPD 的检出率。数据分析常用软件进行，如 RAPDistance Package 分析软件、Popgene 聚类分析软件等。

进行 RAPD 分析时，每个 RAPD – PCR 反应中 DNA 模板的终浓度应控制在 10 – 100ng 范围内。在实际实验中，最佳的模板浓度取决于研究的类群和模板的纯度。此外，不同厂家、不同品牌的 DNA 聚合酶常产生不同 RAPD 产物。因此，在 RAPD – PCR 中不允许实验中途更换 DNA 聚合酶。

三、扩增酶切片段多态性（amplified fragment length polymorphism，AFLP）标记技术

AFLP 标记技术是一种建立在 PCR 技术和 RFLP 技术基础上，利用 PCR 技术扩增 DNA 限制性酶切片段的 DNA 分子标记技术。首先用限制性酶产生基因组 DNA 酶切片段，然后使用双链接头与基因组 DAN 的酶切片段连接形成扩增反应的模板。由于不同物种的基因组 DNA 序列不同，基因组 DNA 经限制性内切酶酶切后产生大小不同的限制性片段。使用特定的双链接头与酶切 DNA 片段连接作为 PCR 的模板，用含有选择性碱基的引物（在引物的 3′端增加 1~3 个核苷酸）对模板 DNA 进行扩增，选择性碱基的种类、数目和顺序决定了扩增的结果。这样，只有那些限制性位点侧翼的核苷酸与引物的选择性碱基相匹配的片段才能被扩增，扩增产物经聚丙烯酰胺凝胶电泳分离、染色，然后根据凝胶上 DNA 指纹的有无来检测物种基因组 DNA 的多态性。在技术特点上，实际上是 RAPD 标记和 RFLP 标记相结合的结果。它结合了 RFLP 和 PCR 技术特点，具有 RFLP 技术的可靠性和 PCR 技术的高效性；并克服了 RAPD 标记稳定性差及标记呈隐性遗传的缺点；同时与 RFLP 比较，用 PCR 技术代替了分子杂交技术，更加方便快捷。由于 AFLP 扩增可使某一品种出现特定的 DNA 谱带，而在另一品种中可能无此谱带产生，因此，这种通过引物诱导及 DNA 扩增后得到的 DNA 多态性可作为一种分子标记。

AFLP 标记原理是对基因组 DNA 限制性酶切片段进行选择性扩增。首先用限制性酶产生基因组 DNA 酶切片段，然后使用双链接头与基因组 DAN 的酶切片段链接形成扩增反应的模板。由于不同物种的基因组 DNA 序列不同，基因组 DNA 经限制性内切酶酶切后产生大小不同的限制性片段。使用特定的双链接头与酶切 DNA 片段连接作为 PCR 的模板，用含有选择性碱基的引物（在引物的 3′端增加 1~3 个核苷酸）对模板 DNA 进行扩增，选择性碱基的种类、数目和顺序决定了扩增的结果。这样，只有那些限制性位点侧翼的核苷酸与引物的选择性碱基相匹配的片段才能被扩增，扩增产物经聚丙烯酰胺凝胶电泳分离、染色，然后根据凝胶上 DNA 指纹的有无来检测物种基因组 DNA 的多态性。

这一技术实验流程主要包括基因组 DNA 的提取和检测、限制性内切酶切割、接头连接、预扩增、选择性 PCR 扩增、凝胶电泳检测和实验数据分析等几个基本步骤。其中，酶切和 PCR 扩增为关键步骤。DNA 模板酶切是否完全会严重影响 AFLP 的结果，同时，DNA 的纯度也是重要的影响因素，因此在 AFLP 标记实验中，PCR 扩增一般分两步进行，第一步为预扩增，预扩增的产物一般稀释 20 倍后作为选择性扩增的模板，预扩增起到了一定的纯化模板的作用。

AFLP 的引物由三部分构成，分别为核心区、酶切位点区和选择性碱基区。核心区序列基本保持不变，酶切位点区与限制性内切酶的酶切位点配对，选择性碱基区通常为 1~3 个碱基，可随机选择。一般带 3 个选择性碱基的引物组合较合适，减少碱基数会使条带过多，不利于统计分析，增加碱基数则会导致条带过少，多态性降低，不能准确鉴定。

四、简单重复序列区间（inter – simple sequence repeat，ISSR）标记技术

ISSR 标记技术是在简单重复序列（simple sequence repeat，SSR）标记技术基础上发展起来的，扩增重复序列之间区域的 DNA 分析技术。在 SSR 序列的 3′端或 5′端加上 2 – 4 个随机核苷酸作为锚定引物，锚定引物可引起特定位点退火，导致与锚定引物互补的间隔不太大的重复序列间 DNA 片段进行 PCR 扩增。扩增产物经聚丙烯酰胺凝胶或者较高浓度的琼脂糖凝胶电泳分离获得扩增指纹图谱。

ISSR 标记技术的操作步骤包括：DNA 的提取及检测、引物设计、PCR 扩增、RCR 产物的电泳检测和实验数据分析。引物设计是 ISSR 标记中最关键的一步，筛选出多态性强、重复性好的引物是整个实验成功的关键。ISSR 引物可参考加拿大 University of British Columbia 所设计的引物。

五、DNA 条形码技术

DNA 条形码（DNA barcoding）技术是利用一个或少数几个标准的 DNA 序列作为标记，对现有的生物物种进行快速、准确的识别和鉴定的一种技术。加拿大奎尔夫大学的 Paul Hebert 教授在 DNA 分类学基础上，对动物界的脊椎动物和无脊椎动物共 11 门 13320 个物种的线粒体细胞色素 C 氧化酶亚基（Cytochrome C oxidase I，COI）基因序列进行分析比较发现，98% 的物种遗传距离差异在种内和种间存在显著差异，其中种内为 0 – 2%，种间平均可达到 11.3%。受条形码技术启发，Hebert 提出可以用单一的小片段基因序列来区分物种，做为物种的条形编码，即 DNA 条形码。DNA 条形码技术通过对一组来自不同生物个体的短的同源 DNA 序列（约 800dp）进行 PCR 扩增和测序，随后对测得的序列进行多重序列比对和聚类分析，从而将某个个体精确定位到一个已描述过的分类群中。但是并不是所有的基因片段都适合作 DNA 条形码，理想的 DNA 条形码应该符合以下条件：

1. 序列的变异幅度要适度。要求在种间的变异幅度要足够大，便于区分不同的物种，同时要具有相对的保守性，确保种内变异相对小而稳定。

2. 必须是用一段标准的 DNA 区域来尽可能鉴别不同的分类群。

3. 序列应当包含足够的系统进化信息以准确定位物种在分类系统中的位置。

4. 应该具有高度保守的引物设计区，以便于设计通用引物进行大规模扩增和测序。

5. 目标 DNA 区应该足够的短。便于 PCR 扩增，尤其是对存在部分 DNA 降解的材料，如存放已久的腊叶标本，处理过的中药药材等，并在现有的技术条件下，可以一次完成测序，DNA 条形码技术的基本操作步骤包括样品取材，提取 DNA，条形码 DNA 序列的扩增与测序，序列对比分析，将结果提交到相关数据库。样品取材时应避免使用发霉或混有其他生物体的材料；来源于动物的药材可以选择 COI 基因，来源于植物的药材可以选择 ITS，martK 和 rbcL 等基因，也可以使用组合片段。

Section 5　DNA Molecular Identification of Crude Drugs

With the development of molecular biology technology，many types of molecular marker identification techniques have been born. The identification of bio – pharmaceutical molecules is based on the polymorphism of biological DNA molecules. It is a new method for the identification of crude drugs by DNA molecular markers to determine their source and evaluate their quality.

Restriction fragment length polymorphism (RFLP) labeling technology

RFLP is the earliest DNA labeling technology, which is a technique to detect allelic variation (polymorphism) of different genetic sites by displaying the size of restriction fragment.

For individual individuals in different populations or populations, there are polymorphism differences in their DNA sequences, which are mainly due to two mutation methods: One is that a single base mutation occurs at the recognition site of restriction endonuclease, which makes the original restriction site disappear or produce new sites; the other is that the length of the restriction fragment changes due to the deletion or insertion of the fragment. When using the same restriction endonuclease to cut the DNA sequences of different species or populations, the length of the restriction fragments varies due to the homology and variation of the target DNA, resulting in different length, size and number of restriction fragments.

At present, RFLP labeling technology is often used in combination with PCR technology. First, the restriction endonuclease recognition sequence containing one or more polymorphisms is amplified by PCR technology, and then the amplified products are cut by the endonuclease and separated by electrophoresis. According to the distribution of restriction fragment length polymorphism, the specificity of different alleles can be judged to achieve the purpose of identification. The PCR – RFLP label allows analysis of trace amounts of DNA samples without sequencing and with less instrumentation limitations. However, primers that can amplify target sequences need to be designed and synthesized beforehand.

Random amplified polymorphic DNA (RAPD) labeling technology

RAPD marker technology is a kind of genetic marker technique based on PCR technology, which can analyze the whole genome polymorphism. This technique often uses random primers for PCR. For DNA of different templates, amplification with the same primer can obtain the same electrophoresis band (high homologous template genome) or different electrophoresis band, so that the polymorphism of template DNA can be reflected by the polymorphism of the same primer amplification band.

The procedure of RAPD is similar to that of PCR, including DNA extraction, purity and concentration detection, PCR amplification, product electrophoresis detection and experimental data analysis. However, a lower annealing temperature such as 36℃ is generally used to ensure stable binding of the primer to the template, while allowing proper mismatching to expand the pairing randomness of the primer in the genomic DNA and increase the detection rate of the RAPD. Data analysis software commonly used, such as RAPDistance Package analysis software, Popgene clustering analysis software.

During RAPD analysis, the final concentration of the DNA template in each RAPD – PCR reaction should be controlled in the range of 10 – 100 ng. In actual experiments, the optimal template concentration depends on the studied taxon and the purity of the template. In addition, DNA polymerases from different manufacturers and brands often produce different RAPD products. Therefore, it is not allowed to replace DNA polymerase in RAPD – PCR.

3. Amplified fragment length polymorphism (AFLP) labeling technology

AFLP labeling technology is a DNA molecular marker technology based on PCR technology and RFLP technology, which uses PCR technology to amplify DNA restriction fragments. First, the genomic DNA fragment was produced by restriction enzyme, and then the fragment of genomic DAN was ligated with double strand junction to form the template of amplification reaction. Due to the different genomic DNA sequences of different species, genomic DNA is digested with restriction endonucleases to produce restriction fragments of different sizes. Use a specific double – linker to ligated with the digested DNA fragment as a template for PCR, and use a primer containing a selective base (add 1 – 3 nucleotides at the 3'end of the primer) to amplify the template DNA. The type, number and order of bases determine the result of the amplification. In this way, only those fragments whose nucleotides flanking the restriction site match the selective base of the primer can be amplified. The amplified products are separated and stained by polyacrylamide gel electrophoresis, and then the polymorphism of DNA is detected according to the presence or absence of DNA fingerprints on the gel.

The experimental procedure of AFLP labeling technology mainly includes several basic steps: extraction and detection of genomic DNA, restriction endonuclease cutting and joint connection, pre – amplification, selective PCR amplification, gel electrophoresis detection and experimental data analysis. Among them, enzymatic digestion and PCR amplification are the key steps. Whether DNA template digestion completely affects the results of AFLP, and the purity of DNA is also an important factor. Therefore, in AFLP labeling experiments, PCR amplification is generally performed in two steps. The first step is pre – amplification. The products of pre – amplification is generally diluted by 20 times and serve as templates for selective amplification. Pre – amplification plays a certain role in purifying templates.

The primers of AFLP are composed of three parts: core region, restriction site region and selective base region. The sequence of the core region remains basically unchanged, and the restriction region is paired with the restriction enzyme site of the selected restriction endonuclease, and the selective base region is usually 1 – 3 bases, which can be randomly selected. Generally, the combination of primers with 3 selective bases is appropriate, and reducing the number of bases will lead to too many bands, which is not conducive to statistical analysis, while increasing the number of bases will lead to too few bands and reduced polymorphism, which cannot be accurately identified.

4. Inter – simple sequence repeat (ISSR) labeling technology

ISSR labeling technology is a DNA analysis technology that amplifies the region between repeated sequences based on the simple repeat sequence (SSR) labeling technology. Adding

2 – 4 random nucleotides as anchor primers at the 3'or 5' end of the SSR sequence. Anchoring primers can cause specific site annealing, resulting in PCR amplification of DNA fragments between repetitive sequences with less complementary spacing to anchored primers. The amplified product was separated by polyacrylamide gel or higher concentration agarose gel to obtain an amplified fingerprint.

The operation steps of ISSR labeling technology include: DNA extraction and detection, primer design, PCR amplification, electrophoresis detection of RCR products and experimental data analysis. Primer design is the most critical step in ISSR labeling. Screening for primers with strong polymorphism and good reproducibility is the key to the success of the whole experiment. ISSR primers can be referenced to primers designed by the University of British Columbia, Canada.

5. DNA barcode technology

DNA barcoding technology is a technique that uses one or a few standard DNA sequences as markers to quickly and accurately identify and identify existing biological species. On the basis of DNA taxonomy, Professor Paul Hebert of Guelphin University, Canada, analyzed and compared the mitochondrial Cytochrome C oxidase I (COI) subgroup gene sequences of 11 phyla, 13320 species of vertebrates and invertebrates in animal kingdom. It was found that 98% of the genetic distances of species were significantly different within and between species. The average intraspecific and interspecific rates were 0 – 2% and 11. 3% respectively. Inspired by barcode technology, Hebert proposed that a single small fragment of gene sequence can be used to distinguish species as a bar coding of species, which is DNA barcode.

DNA barcode technology can accurately locate an individual to a described taxonomic group by PCR amplifying and sequencing a group of short homologous DNA sequences (about 800dp) from different organisms, and then performing multiple sequence alignment and clustering analysis on the measured sequences. However, not all gene fragments are suitable for DNA barcoding. The ideal DNA barcoding should meet the following conditions:

The variation of the sequence should be moderate. It is required that the variation range between species should be large enough to distinguish different species, and at the same time be relatively conservative, ensuring that intraspecific variation is relatively small and stable.

A standard DNA region must be used to identify as many different taxa as possible.

3. The sequence should contain sufficient phylogenetic information to accurately locate the species in the classification system.

4. It should have a highly conserved primer design area to facilitate the design of universal primers for large – scale amplification and sequencing.

5. The target DNA region should be short enough. It is convenient for PCR amplification, especially for materials with partial DNA degradation, such as long – lasting wax specimens, treated Chinese herbal medicines, etc. , and can be sequenced once under the existing technical conditions.

The basic operation steps of DNA barcode technology include sampling, DNA extraction, amplification and sequencing of barcode DNA sequences, sequence comparison analysis, and submission of results to relevant databases. Avoid using moldy or mixed materials with other organisms when sampling; the animal – derived herbs can be selected from the COI gene, and the plant – derived herbs can be selected from genes such as ITS, martK and rbcL, or combined fragments.

第二章 实验内容

Chapter Two Experimental Contents

实验一 植物细胞、细胞后含物的观察及藻、菌类生药的鉴定

【实验目的】

1. 掌握 藻、菌类生药的鉴定方法；水装片和透化法装片的制作方法。

2. 了解 显微镜的构造、使用及保养方法；植物细胞的结构特征，掌握植物细胞后含物的显微特征；藻类、菌类的主要特征，识别常见药用藻类和菌类。

【实验材料】

1. **新鲜材料** 洋葱鳞茎、马铃薯块茎。

2. **原植物蜡叶标本** 海带、昆布、羊栖菜、海蒿子。

3. **药材及饮片** 冬虫夏草、灵芝、茯苓、猪苓。

4. **生药粉末** 天花粉、大黄、半夏、甘草、黄柏、茯苓、猪苓、灵芝孢子、马勃。

【实验仪器与试剂】

1. **仪器** 显微镜、载玻片、盖玻片、单面刀片、镊子、酒精灯、纱布、小玻棒、擦镜纸、吸水纸、电水浴、试管、坩埚、试管夹。

2. **试剂** 稀甘油、蒸馏水、5%氢氧化钾试液、碘化钾－碘试液。

【实验内容】

一、植物细胞的观察

取载玻片，在中央部位滴加蒸馏水一滴，用镊子撕取洋葱鳞叶内表皮一小块（2~3 mm²）放在水滴上，将盖玻片一边触及液滴边缘，轻轻放下盖玻片，不要产生气泡，流溢于盖玻片以外及上部的水必须用吸水纸吸去。置于显微镜下观察。

观察要点：细胞的形态、构造。

二、细胞后含物的观察

1. 淀粉粒

（1）取载玻片，在中央部位滴加蒸馏水一滴，用单面刀片切开马铃薯块茎外皮、刮取浆液少许，溶在蒸馏水中，盖上盖玻片，置于显微镜下观察。

（2）取天花粉粉末少许，用蒸馏水装片，置于显微镜下观察。

观察要点：淀粉粒的形状、大小、类型（单粒、复粒、半复粒），脐点的形状、位置。

2. **草酸钙结晶** 分别取大黄、甘草、半夏粉末少许，放在不同的载玻片中央，加水合氯醛1滴，用小玻棒搅匀，在酒精灯上微微加热至近沸腾，可随时补加水合氯醛，避免蒸干。稍冷，滴加稀甘油1滴，搅拌均匀（透化），加盖玻片，置显微镜下观察。

观察要点：草酸钙结晶的形态、大小、存在部位。

三、藻类、菌类生药的形态特征

1. 昆布（海带、昆布）、海藻（羊栖菜、海蒿子）腊叶标本的观察。

2. 冬虫夏草、灵芝、茯苓、猪苓药材标本的观察。

四、菌类生药的显微鉴定

1. **茯苓粉末的观察** 取茯苓粉末少许，分别用蒸馏水及5%氢氧化钾液装片，置显微镜下观察。

观察要点如下。

水装片：无色颗粒状团块或末端钝圆的分枝状团块。

5%氢氧化钾液装片：可见菌丝，细长，稍弯曲，有分枝，无色（内部菌丝）或带棕色（外层菌丝），横壁偶见（图2-1）。

2. **猪苓粉末的观察** 取猪苓粉末少许，用蒸馏水装片，置显微镜下观察。

观察要点：菌丝团无色（内部菌丝）或棕色（外层菌丝），菌丝

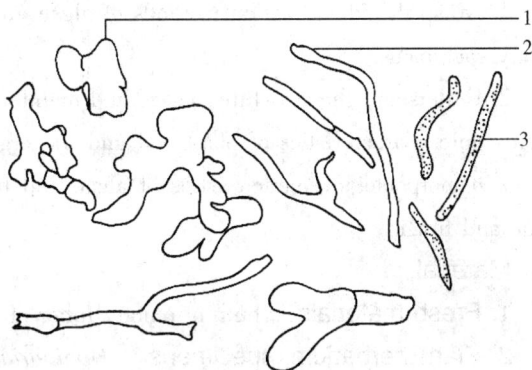

图2-1 茯苓粉末
1. 分枝状团块 2. 无色菌丝 3. 棕色菌丝

细长，弯曲，有分枝或结节状膨大，无色或棕色，草酸钙结晶呈双锥形或八面体形。

3. **马勃粉末的观察** 取马勃粉末少许，用蒸馏水装片，置显微镜下观察。

观察要点：孢丝、孢子的形态、表面情况、草酸钙方晶。

五、理化鉴定

茯苓、猪苓的鉴定 分别取茯苓、猪苓粉末少许于试管中，加碘化钾-碘试液数滴，观察溶液颜色，比较其实验结果的差异。

【报告要求】

1. 绘洋葱鳞叶表皮细胞图，并注明各部位名称。

2. 绘马铃薯及天花粉的淀粉粒图，比较它们的不同，并注明各部位名称。

3. 绘大黄、半夏、甘草草酸钙结晶图，并注明结晶类型。

4. 绘茯苓、猪苓、马勃的粉末组织构造图。

5. 记录茯苓、猪苓的理化鉴定操作及结果。

【思考题】

1. 植物细胞后含物的观察方法有哪些？在生药鉴定中的意义是什么？

2. 藻类植物有哪些共同特征？菌类植物有哪些共同特征？比较藻、菌类植物形态的异同点。

3. 什么是菌核、菌丝体、子座和子实体？

4. 茯苓与猪苓在性状、显微特征上有哪些异同点？

Experiment 1　Observation of Plant Cells and Their Ergastic Substances and Identification of Algae and Fungi Crude Drugs

Aim

1. Grasp the identification methods of algae and fungi. Grasp the methods of making temporary specimens.

2. Understand the structure, usage and maintenance of optical microscope. Understand the microscopic characteristics of plant cell and the ergastic substances in plant cells. Understand the main morphologic characteristics of algae and fungi; identify the common pharmaceutical algae and fungi.

Material

1. Fresh materials　bulb of onion, tuber of potato.

2. Plant herbarium specimens　*Laminaria japonica*, Ecklonia kurome, Sargassum fusiforme *and* Sargassum pallidum.

3. Crude drugs and their proceeded products　Dongchongxiacao (Chinese caterpilar fungus), Lingzhi (lucid ganoderma), Fuling (Indian bread), Zhuling (polyporus) .

4. Powders　Tianhuafen (snakegourd root), Dahuang (rhubarb), Banxia (pinellia tuber), Gancao (licorice root), Fuling (Indian bread), Zhuling (polyporus), Lingzhi (spore of ganoderma), Mabo (puffball) .

Equipment and reagents

1. Optical microscope, slide, cover glass, one side blade, nippers, alcohol lamp, gauze, glass stick, lens paper, absorbent paper, hydroelectric bath, test tube, melting pot and tube clip.

2. Dilute glycerine, distilled water, 5% potassium hydroxide solution, potassium iodide – iodine solution.

Methods

1. The observation of plant cells

Add one drop of distilled water in a slide center, tear off a bit of endepidermis ($2-3\ mm^2$) of an onion scale leaf with nipper, put it into that water and take one side of cover glass to touch the liquid surface and lay down the cover glass without making any bubble. The water over the cover glass must be absorbed by absorbent paper and then observe the slide under microscope.

Main points of observation: form and structure of cells.

2. The observation of ergastic substances in plant cells

(1) Starch grains

① Add one drop of distilled water in a slide center, scrape off a bit of liquid on the cut surface of potato with one side blade and put it into the water, cover with a cover glass and observe under microscope.

② Take a bit of powder of snakegourd root, mount with water and observe.

Main points of observation: form, size and type (simple grain, compound grain, half – compound grain) of starch grains; form and position of hilar spot.

(2) Calcium oxalate crystals   Add one drop of chloral hydratein a slide centre, take a bit of powder of rhubarb, licorice root and pinellia tuber by a glass stick separately, mix with one drop of chloral hydrate and heat the slide near to boiling on alcohol lamp. Add chloral hydrate in any time in order to prevent from dryness by evaporation. After it becomes cooled, add one drop of dilute glycerine and mix uniformly, then cover with a cover glass and observe coverslip and test under microscope.

Main points of observation: the form and size ofalcium oxalate crystals.

3. Morphologic characteristics of algae and fungi crude drugs

(1) Thallus laminariae (*Laminaria japonica*, *Ecklonia kurome*), thallus sargassi (*Sargassum fusiforme*, *Sargassum pallidum*).

(2) Chinese caterpilar fungus, ganoderma, Indian bread, and polyporus.

4. Microscopic identification of fungi crude drugs

(1) Observation of Indian bread powder   Take a bit of Indian bread powder, mount with water or 5% potassium hydroxide solution and observe under microscope.

Main points of observation after mounting with water: colorless granulo – clumping or cladodromous clumping with blunt ends.

Mount with 5% potassium hydroxide solution: slender, colorless or brown, slightly bent hypha with branch andhypha with cross walls occasionally.

(2) Observation of polyporus powder   Take a bit of polyporus powder, mount with water or 5% potassium hydroxide solution and observe under microscope. Main points of observation: colorless (internal hypha) or brown (external hypha) hypha clump and double cones or octahedron shape of calcium oxalate crystals.

(3) Observation of puffball powder   Take a bit of puffball powder, mount with water or 5% potassium hydroxide solution and observe under microscope. Main points of observation: capillitia, the shape and state on surface of spore and square crystals of calcium oxalate.

5. Identification of Indian bread and polyporus with physical and chemical method

Take a little of powder of Indian bread and polyporus, into test tube, add potassium iodide – iodine solution into powder, observe the solution color and compare the different results between two kinds of powder.

Points in experiment report

1. Draw the diagram of epidermic cells of the onion scale leaf and sign the names of each part.

2. Draw the diagrams of starch grains of potato and snakegourd root and sign the names of each part.

3. Draw the diagrams of calcium oxalate crystals of rhubarb, pinellia tuber and licorice root and sign the type of crystals.

4. Draw the diagrams of microscopic characteristics of powdered Indian bread, polyporus and puffball.

5. Record the operation and results of physical and chemical identification of Indian bread and polyporus.

Topics for thinking

1. What are the observation methods of the ergastic substances in plant cells? What are the significances of the ergastic substances for crude drugs identification?

2. What are the common morphologic characteristics of algae and fungi? Compare their similarities and differences of appearance between algae and fungi?

3. What are sclerotium, hypha, stroma and sporophore?

4. What are the similarities and differences of appearance and microscopic characteristics between Indian bread and polyporus?

实验二　植物的组织构造

【实验目的】

1. 掌握　植物六大组织的形态、构造与功能。
2. 熟悉　各种组织在植物体内的主要分布位置。

【实验材料】

1. **新鲜材料**　薄荷叶、洋地黄叶、菘蓝叶、蒲公英根、曼陀罗叶。
2. **药材**　肉桂、厚朴、苦杏仁、生姜。
3. **石蜡切片**　洋葱根尖、薄荷茎、接骨木、厚朴、陈皮、松枝茎、南瓜茎。

【实验仪器与试剂】

1. **仪器**　显微镜、载玻片、盖玻片、单面刀片、镊子、酒精灯、纱布、小玻棒、擦镜纸、吸水纸。
2. **试剂**　稀甘油、水合氯醛、蒸馏水、间苯三酚、稀盐酸、苏丹Ⅲ试液、20%醋酸溶液。

【实验内容】

一、分生组织

（一）初生分生组织

取洋葱根尖纵切面制片，置于低倍镜观察，可见在根尖的先端有许多排列疏松的细胞群组成一个帽状的根冠，内侧就是根的顶端分生组织。

根据下列几个方面仔细观察其形态结构：

（1）细胞壁的性状。
（2）细胞壁的厚薄。
（3）细胞质的稀稠。
（4）细胞核与细胞体积的比例。
（5）细胞排列的情况。
（6）细胞与细胞之间有无间隙存在。

（二）次生分生组织

1. **形成层**　取薄荷茎横切片，置于显微镜下观察，可见排列成环状的维管束，在维管束的木质部（在切片中，被染成红色细胞的所在部位）与韧皮部（与前者相对一端，被染成深绿色的一群细胞）之间，可见排列整齐，紧密略呈扁长方形的细胞群，这就是形成层。

2. **木栓形成层**　取接骨木横切片，置于显微镜下观察，可见规则排列的几行木栓细胞。木栓细胞的特点是扁平形、径壁吻合、褐色且无细胞间隙。在木栓细胞下的一层含有原生质体，并处于分裂状态的活细胞，被称为木栓形成层。木栓细胞形成层——切向（即平行于表皮的）横壁分裂，所以往外产生栓化的、死细胞，而向内则产生栓化的、饱含着活的原生质体的细胞（栓内层细胞）。

由已栓化的木栓细胞、木栓形成层和栓内层细胞共同组成复杂的保护组织——周皮。

二、保护组织

（一）初生保护组织

1. **表皮细胞与气孔器**　用镊子撕去所备植物叶的下表皮一小片，用水装片，于显微镜下观察，注意表皮细胞的形状和排列有何特点？在这些表皮细胞之间分布着一些由二个半月形的保卫细胞组成的气孔，注意保卫细胞和副卫细胞之间的联系，并说出它是哪种类型气孔。

2. **毛茸**　用镊子撕取洋地黄叶表皮或叶柄表皮一小片，用水装片，于显微镜下观察，可见在表皮细胞上长有多细胞的先端尖锐的毛茸，即为非腺毛。此外，再仔细观察，可见有些毛茸，先端不呈尖锐状，而有类圆球状的头部与短柱状柄部之分的，即为腺毛。注意洋地黄叶腺毛的头部和柄部各由多少细胞组成。

3. **角质层**　取薄荷茎横切片，于显微镜下观察，可见最外面的一层细胞，排列紧密并且整齐，即为表皮细胞的横切面观，然后转换高倍镜，可见表皮细胞外侧有一层折光较强的角质层。

（二）次生保护组织

1. 木栓组织侧面观（横切面） 取厚朴树皮横切片，于显微镜下观察，可见厚朴的最外侧有数层排列整齐，长方形的细胞即为木栓组织的侧面观。

2. 木栓组织的顶面观 用刀片纵向刮取厚朴树皮表面的木栓组织少许，用水合氯醛装片，于显微镜下观察，可见多数淡黄棕色，成多角形的细胞，即为木栓组织的顶面观。

三、基本组织与机械组织

1. 基本组织 观察薄荷茎横切面的厚角组织之后，注意位于厚角组织两侧以及茎的最中央有许多类圆形的薄壁细胞，细胞与细胞之间有明显的间隙，该细胞群即为基本组织。

2. 厚角组织 取薄荷茎横切片，于显微镜下观察，可见茎四角处的表皮层之内，有一群细胞，其角隅处的细胞壁特别增厚，该细胞群即为厚角组织。

3. 厚壁组织——纤维、石细胞 取肉桂粉末少许（或直接取肉桂片段，用刀片刮取粉末），以水合氯醛装片，置于显微镜下观察，可见某些细胞呈长梭形，细胞壁很厚，胞腔很小或看不清胞腔，这种细胞即为纤维。

用镊子撕取苦杏仁种皮一小片，以水合氯醛装片，进行观察，可见多数散在的黄色类圆形石细胞，其细胞壁增厚，并有许多纹孔。

石细胞、纤维的细胞壁木质化，遇间苯三酚和浓盐酸试液显红色。

四、输导组织

1. 管胞 取松枝茎纵切面切片，于显微镜下观察，可见众多两端斜尖的长梭形管状细胞，即为管胞。高倍镜下在细胞壁上可见到排列成串的圆圈，每个大圆圈就是一个具缘纹孔，调节微调节螺旋，还可见到松枝茎的具缘纹孔有三个同心圆。思考这是什么原因？另外再尽可能找一找具缘纹孔的侧面观。

2. 导管与筛管 取南瓜茎纵切片，于显微镜下观察，可见被番红染料染成红色的长管状组织，即为导管群，注意观察南瓜茎有几种纹理的导管，上下两个导管细胞（导管节）之间有横隔吗？再于导管群两侧观察被亮绿染料染成绿色的薄壁性纵行连接的管状组织，即为筛管群，注意上下两个筛管细胞（筛管节）相接的横隔上有何特征？该横隔就是筛板。

五、分泌组织

1. 分泌细胞 切取生姜一薄片，用水装片，于显微镜下观察，可见椭圆形的细胞，充满黄色溶液，该细胞即为油细胞，黄色溶液即为挥发油。滴加苏丹Ⅲ试液，油液呈红色。

2. 分泌腔 取陈皮横切片，于显微镜下观察，可见有许多薄壁细胞围拢而成的大型圆形腔隙，腔内有残余的细胞壁存在，该腔隙即为分泌腔。

陈皮的分泌腔内含有挥发油，因此又可称为油室。

3. **分泌道** 取松枝茎横切片，于显微镜下观察，可见基本组织中有许多圆形的腔隙，它是由许多分泌细胞围拢形成的管道即为分泌道的横切面，分泌道腔隙内含有树脂，故又可称为树脂道。

4. **乳汁管** 用刀片切取蒲公英根纵向薄片，放在载玻片上，滴加20%醋酸一滴，微热后，加苏丹Ⅲ试液数滴，再微微加热，然后加盖玻片，在显微镜下观察，乳汁管内的乳汁被染成红色。

【实验报告】

1. 简述各类组织的形态和功能。

2. 绘出薄荷叶、洋地黄叶、菘蓝叶的气孔，注明各部分的名称。

3. 绘出肉桂的纤维、苦杏仁的石细胞，注明各部分的名称。

4. 绘出生姜的分泌细胞、陈皮的油室及蒲公英的乳汁管。

【思考题】

1. 分生组织中的细胞形态特点是什么？

2. 气孔的作用是什么？具缘纹孔是如何形成的？

Experiment 2 Botanic Tissue Structures

Aim

1. Learn appearance, structures and functions of six kinds of botanic tissue.

2. Familiar with distribution of various botanic tissues.

Material

1. **Fresh materials** leaves of wind mint, Yangdihuangye (foxglove leaves), songlanye (isatis tinctoria) and Pugongyingye (dandelion root), Mantuotuoye (stramonium leaves)

2. **Crude drugs** Rougui (cinnamon bark), Houpu (magnolia bark), Kuxingren (bitter apricot seed) and Jiang (ginger)

3. **Paraffin sections** root tip of onion, stem of wild mint, Jiegumu stem (elder), magnolia bark, Chenpi (orange peel), stem of pine and Nanguajing (stem of pumpkin)

Equipment and reagents

1. Microscope, slide, cover glass, blade, nippers, alcohol lamp, gauze, glass stick, lens paper, absorbent paper

2. Dilute glycerine, chloral hydrate, distilled water, 1, 3, 5 – trihydroxybenzene, dilute hydrochloric acid, Sudan Ⅲ solution, 20% acetic acid solution.

Methods

1. Meristem

（1）Primary meristem Take a piece of a longitudinal section of onion root tip to make a temporary slide, observe under lower power lens, there are many porously arranged cell mass to form a cap shape of root crown, apical meristem is inside.

Observe theappearance and structure in the following aspects:

① Description of cell wall;

② Thickness of cell wall;

③ Denseness of cytoplasm;

④ Ratio of caryon to cell volume;

⑤ Arrangement of cells;

⑥ Existence of interspace between cells.

（2）Secondary meristem

① Cambium　Take a cross section of wind mint stem; test under microscope. Circular vascular bundles can be seen, cambium is between xylem（the red – dyed part in cross section）and phloem（the green – dyed cells opposite to xylem）in vascular bundle, which is a rectangle cell mass arranged in order and tightly.

② Phellogen　Take a cross section of elder stem, test under microscope. We can see several raws of flat, brown cork cell arranged in order, with coinciding longitudinal walls and without cell spaces; beneath the cork cells, a layer of living cells contained protoplast are in division state, so the layer is called phellogen; phellogen cells split along tangent walls（parallel to epidermal）, so that they generate suberized dead cells outside, and nonsuberized cells with live protoplast（phelloderm cells）inside.

Periderm is the complicated protective tissue composed by suberized cork cells, phellogen and phelloderm.

2. Protective tissue

（1）Primary protective tissues

① Epidermic cells and stomatal apparatus　Tear a tablet of the prepared leaves, mount with water and test under microscope, pay attention to shape and arrangement characteristics of epidermic cells. Stoma, composed of two semilunate guard cells, distributes among some of epidermic cells. Pay attention to the relationship of guard cells and accessory cells and what type the stoma belongs to.

② Pappo　Tear a tablet of epidermis or petiol epidermis of foxglove leaves, mount with water and test under microscope and we can see pappo with shape apex on epidermic cells, which is called nonglandular hair. Besides, some pappo, whose apex is not sharp but with subsphaeroidal head or stub like petiole, is called glandular hair. Pay attention to the cell number of glandular head and petiole of foxglove leaves.

③ Cuticulum　Take a cross section of mild mint stem and test under microscope, the outermost layer of cells arranges regularly and compactly, which is the cross section view of epidermis. Then switch to high power lens and we can see the layer of cuticulum with strong refraction outside the epidermis.

（2）Secondary protective tissue

① Lateral view of cork tissue（cross section）   Test a cross section of magnolia bark un-der microscope and we can see the outermost several layers of brick – shaped cells arranged regularly.

② Apical view of cork tissue   Tear a bit of cork tissue from epidermis of magnolia bark longitudinally with blade, mount with chloral hydrate and test under microscope and we can see many light yellowish – brown and polygonal cells.

3. Elementary tissue and mechanical tissue

（1）Elementary tissue   When we observe the collenchyma in cross section of mild mint stem, pay attention to the many subrotund parenchyma cells located on two sides of collenchy-ma and in stem center, and the interspace between cells is obvious, which cell mass is elemen-tary tissue.

（2）Collenchyma   Test a cross section of mild mint stem under microscope and we can see the cell mass in epidermis on four corners of stem with extraordinarily thick walls in cor-ners, which cell masse are called collenchyma.

（3）Sclerenchyma—fibers and stone cells   Take a bit of powder of cinnamon bark, mount with chloral hydrate and test under microscope, we can see some fusiform cells with thick wall and small or unclear cell lumen and these cells are called fibers.

Tear a tablet of testa of bitter apricot seed, mount with chloral hydrate and test under mi-croscope; we can see the scattered yellow subrotund stone cells with thick walls and many pits. The walls of stone cells and fibers are lignified and they can become red when they meet 1, 3, 5 – trihydroxybenzene and concentrated hydrochloric acid.

4. Conducting tissue

（1）Tracheids   Test a longitudinal section of pine stem under microscope, many fusiform tubiform cells with cuspidal end called tracheid can be seen. Under high powder lens, we can see bunchy rings arranged regularly on the cell walls, each big circle is a bordered pit, and three concentric circles are found by regulating fine adjusting screw, why? Further, look for the lateral view of bordered pits as far as possible.

（2）Vessels and sieve tubes   Test a longitudinal section of pumpkin stem under micro-scope and the red tubiform tissue dyed by safranine called vessel mass can be found. Pay atten-tion to types of vessel texture and whether there is saeptum between two longitudinal – connect-ed vessel cells. The tubiform tissue dyed into green on both sides of vessel mass is longitudinal – connected sieve tubes with thin walls and the septum between two longitudinal – connected sieve tubes is sieve plate.

5. Secretory tissue

（1）Secretory cells   Cut a slice of ginger, mount with water and test under microscope, elliptic cells full of yellow solution are called secretory cells and the yellow solution is volatile oil. The oil shows red as Sudan III solution is droped in.

（2）Secretory cavities　Test a cross section of orange peel under microscope and the large round lacounas surrounded by many parenchyma cells called secretory cavity can be found, in which, some rqliq cell walls are left.

Due tovolatile oil contained in secretory cavity of orange peel, so they are also called oil cavity.

（3）Secretory canals　Test a cross section of pine stem under microscope and we can see many rounded lacounas in elementary tissue, which are cross sections of tubular secretory canals formed by many secretory cells. The lacounas of secretory canals contain resin in pine stem, so they are called resin canals.

（4）Laticiferous vessels　Cut a longitudinal section of dandelion root, put on a slide, add a drop of 20% acetic acid and heat gently, add several drops of Sudan III solution and then heat gently again, cover with a coverslip and test under microscope, the milk in laticiferous vessels is dyed red.

Points in experiment report

1. State the property and functions of each type of tissue simply.

2. Draw the stoma of wild mint leaves, foxglove leaves and isatis tinctoria leaves and sign the names of each part.

3. Draw fibers of cinnamon bark and stone cells of bitter apricot seed and sign the names of each part.

4. Draw secretory cells of ginger, oil cavities of orange peel and lactifers of dandelion.

Topics for thinking

1. What are the morphologic characteristics of the cells in the meristem?

2. What are the functions of stoma? How the bordered pits form?

实验三　根类生药的组织构造

【实验目的】

1. 掌握　双子叶植物根的初生构造、次生构造、异常构造及单子叶植物根的构造，比较其异同点。

2. 了解　根类药材的性状鉴定方法。

3. 识别植物根的性状特征，了解变态根的形态特征及种类。

【实验材料】

1. **新鲜材料**　桔梗、芍药、板蓝根、天门冬、吊兰、龟背竹等植物的根。

2. **根类药材**　何首乌、川牛膝、乌头及附子、白头翁、白芍、赤芍、板蓝根、地榆、黄芪、人参、三七、白芷、独活、柴胡、党参、防风、防己、龙胆、丹参、黄芩、茜草、玄参、地黄、沙参、苦参、桔梗、麦冬、天门冬、郁金、当归、百部。

3. **石蜡切片**　细辛根、芍药根、牛膝根、百部根的横切片。

4. 药材粉末 黄芩、白芍、桔梗。

【实验仪器与试剂】

1. 仪器 光学显微镜、载玻片、盖玻片、单面刀片、镊子、酒精灯、培养皿、纱布、小玻棒、擦镜纸、滤纸条、试管（10 ml）、小玻璃漏斗。

2. 试剂 水合氯醛试液、稀甘油、蒸馏水、间苯三酚、浓盐酸。

【实验内容】

一、根的外部形态与变态种类

观察新鲜桔梗、芍药、板蓝根、天门冬、吊兰、龟背竹等植物根的外部形态，辨别根的变态种类。

二、根类药材的性状鉴定

观察何首乌、川牛膝、乌头及附子、白头翁、白芍、赤芍、板蓝根、地榆、黄芪、三七、白芷、独活、柴胡、党参、防风、防己、龙胆、丹参、黄芩、茜草、玄参、地黄、沙参、苦参、桔梗、麦冬、天门冬、郁金、当归、百部的药材性状。

观察要点：注意形态、大小、色泽、表面、质地、断面、气味等特征。

三、根的内部构造观察

1. 双子叶植物根的初生构造 取细辛根的横切片置显微镜下，由外向内观察（图2-2）。

观察要点：其由外向内的构造如下。

（1）**表皮** 为最外层细胞，排列较整齐。其外壁不角质化，可见表皮细胞向外突出形成的根毛。

（2）**皮层** 位于表皮以内，占根的大部分，又可分为三层：①外皮层：紧靠表皮下方，略呈切向延长的一层细胞；②中皮层：介于外皮层和内皮层之间，排列疏松的多层薄壁细胞；③内皮层：皮层最内层，为排列紧密的一层细胞，可见凯氏点（被染成红色）。

（3）**中柱** 内皮层以内的部分。①中柱鞘：与内皮层相邻，为中柱的最外一层细胞。②木质部：为四原型，由导管、木纤维、木薄壁细胞组成。导管为多角形、壁稍增厚、被染成红色的较大的细胞。③韧皮部：位于木质部星角之间，由筛管、伴胞、韧皮纤维、韧皮薄壁细胞组成。细胞大小不一，被染成蓝色。

2. 单子叶植物根的构造 取百部根的横切片，置显微镜下，由外向内观察。

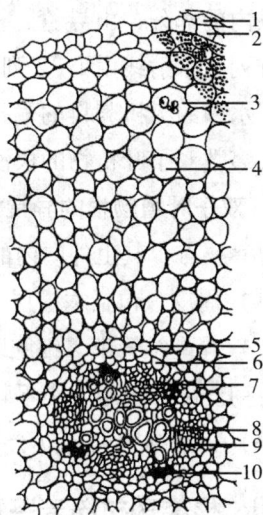

图2-2 北细辛（根）横切面
1. 表皮 2. 下皮 3. 油细胞
4. 皮层 5. 内皮层 6. 中柱鞘
7. 韧皮部 8. 后生木质部
9. 形成层 10. 原生木质部

观察要点：其内部构造如下。

（1）根被　最外面的3～4列细胞，略呈多角形。

（2）皮层　①外皮层：由一层排列紧密的细胞组成；②皮层：占根的大部分，细胞较小；③内皮层：皮层最内的一列排列紧密的细胞，具凯氏点。

（3）中柱　①中柱鞘：位于内皮层内侧，是中柱的外层细胞，由1～2列小型的、切向延长的薄壁细胞组成；②木质部；③韧皮部

3. 双子叶植物根的次生构造　取芍药根的横切片，置显微镜下，由外向内观察。

观察要点：其由外向内的构造如下。

（1）周皮　由木栓层、木栓形成层、栓内层组成，形成双子叶植物根的次生保护组织，具有保护作用。①木栓层：由数列排列整齐的长方形的木栓细胞组成；②木栓形成层：位于木栓层的下方，由中柱鞘细胞恢复分生能力所形成；③栓内层：为数列大型薄壁细胞。一般不含叶绿体，栓内层发达者有"次生皮层"之称。

（2）维管束　由韧皮部、形成层、木质部组成。①韧皮部：位于形成层的外侧，细胞排列较紧密。由筛管、伴胞、韧皮薄壁细胞、韧皮纤维组成。是植物体中输送光合作用制造的有机营养物质到其他部分的输导组织。②形成层：为排列紧密的扁平细胞组成。具有分生能力，向内分生次生木质部，向外分生次生韧皮部。③木质部：形成层以内的部分，由导管、木纤维、木薄壁细胞组成。导管染成红色，大小不一，放射状排列。木射线由1～2列薄壁细胞组成，呈放射状。是植物体中自下而上输送水分及溶于水中的无机养料的输导组织。④射线：位于维管束之间的薄壁细胞，放射状排列。大多数双子叶植物的根没有髓部。

4. 双子叶植物根的异常构造　取牛膝根的横切片，置显微镜下观察。

观察要点：其由外向内的构造如下。

（1）周皮　包括木栓层、木栓形成层、栓内层，但木栓形成层与栓内层不易辨认。

（2）异型维管束　细胞壁染成红色的为导管，是木质部组成的主要部分。木质部外侧为韧皮部，细胞大小不整齐。这些异型维管束呈同心环状排列。

（3）正常维管束　位于中心，为二原型。

四、根类药材粉末鉴定

取黄芩、白芍、桔梗药材粉末，用水合氯醛透化后，稀甘油装片，置显微镜下观察导管、草酸钙结晶、菊糖、乳管、木纤维、木栓细胞等形态特征（图2-3、2-4）。

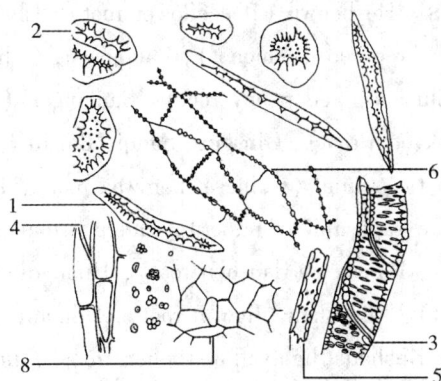

图 2-3　黄芩粉末

1. 韧皮纤维　2. 石细胞　3. 导管

4. 木薄壁细胞　5. 木纤维　6. 韧皮薄壁细胞

7. 淀粉粒　8. 木栓细胞

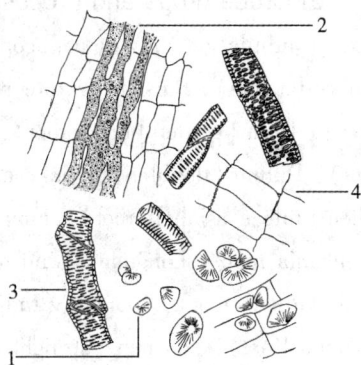

图 2-4　桔梗粉末

1. 菊糖　2. 乳汁管　3. 导管

4. 木薄壁细胞

【报告要求】

1. 描述白芍、赤芍、黄芩、百部的药材性状特征。

2. 绘制细辛、芍药、牛膝、百部根的组织构造简图，标清各组织构造部位的名称。

3. 绘制黄芩、白芍、桔梗粉末特征图，标清各部分显微特征的名称。

【思考题】

1. 常见的变态根有几种？

2. 双子叶植物根的初生构造和次生构造有何主要的不同点？次生构造是如何形成的？

3. 双子叶植物根的初生构造和单子叶植物根的构造有何异同点？

4. 何为根的异常构造？常见的有几种？

5. 白芍和赤芍生药材有哪些主要区别？

Experiment 3　The Microscopic Construction of the Root
Type of Crude Drugs

Aim

1. Learn the primary, secondary and abnormal construction of dicotyledon roots, and the root structure of monocotyledon. Compare the similarities and differences between them.

2. Understand the identifying methods of roots with morphologic characteristics.

3. Discriminate the morphologic characteristics and varieties of vegetable roots and learn morphologic characteristics and varieties of abnormal roots.

Material

1. Fresh root materials　Jiegeng (balloon flower root), Shaoyao (paeony root), Banlangen (isatis root), Tianmendong (lucid asparagus), Diaolan and GuiBeizhu.

2. Crude drugs and processed medicines   Heshouwu（fleeceflower root）, Chuanniuxi（cyathula root）, Wutou（aconite root）, fuzi（prepared commonot）, Baitouweng（Chinese pulsatilla root）, Baishao（white peony root）, Chishao（red peony root）, Banlangen（isatis root）, Diyu（garden burnet root）, Huangqi（milkvetch root）, Ginseng, Sanqi, Baizhi（pai－chi）, Duhuo（doubleteeth pubescent angelica root）, Caihu（Chinese thorowax root）, Dangshen（pilose asiabell root）, Fangfeng（divaricate saposhnikovia root）, Fangji（fourstamen stephania root）, Longdan（Chinese gentian root）, Danshen（danshen root）, Huangqin（baical skullcap root）, Qiancao（Indian madder root）, Xuanshen（figwort root）, Dihuang（rehmannia Root）, Shashen（straight ladybell root）, Kushen（lightyellow sophora root）, Jiegeng（balloon flower root）, Maidong（dwarf lilyturf root）, Tianmendong（lucid asparagus）, Yujin（turmeric root－tuber）, Danggui（Chinese angelica）, Baibu（stemona root）.

3. Root paraffin sections   Xixin（Chinese wild ginger）, Shaoyao（peony root）, Niuxi（achyranthis）and Baibu（stemona root）.

4. Powders   Huangqin（baical skullcap root）, Baishao（white peony root）, Jiegeng（balloon flower root）.

Equipment and reagents

1. Optical microscope, glass slide, cover glass, single plane blade, nippers, alcohol lamp, culture capsule, absorbent gauze, glass stick, lens paper, filter－paper, sample tube and glass funnel.

2. Chloral hydrate solution, dilute glycerin, distilled water, 1, 3, 5－trihydroxybenzene and concentrated hydrochloric acid.

Methods

1. Observe the appearance of all fresh root materials

Observe the appearance of all fresh root materials above and distinguish the varieties of abnormal roots.

2. Appearance identification of all root type of crude drugs above

Main points of observation: shape, size, color and luster, surface, texture, cross－section, odor, etc.

3. Observation of internal constructionof roots

（1）Primary structure of dicotyledon root（the cross section of asarum root）

Main points of observation on theecto－entad structures are as follows:

①Epidermis: It is the outer layer of regularly arranging cells with no keratinized wall and root hair.

②Cortex: It includes the majority in the root cells under the epidermis and is divided into three layers:

Ⅰ. Exodermis: It is a layer of cells extend in tangential direction and is situated closely to the epidermis.

Ⅱ. Mesodermis: It includes the multilayer of loosely arranging parenchyma cells, situated between the exodermis and endodermis.

Ⅲ. Endodermis: It is the innermost layer of closely arranging cells in cortex, in which Casparian dots (dyed into red) can be seen.

③Stele: It is the portion inside the endodermis and is divided into three parts:

Ⅰ. Pericycle: It is the outer layer of stele cells, bordered upon the endodermis.

Ⅱ. Xylem: It is tetrarch and made up of bigger polygon vessels with walls dyed into red, wood fiber and wood parenchyma.

Ⅲ. Phloem: It includes the cell masses dyed into blue in different size, between the stellate xylem and is made up of sieve vessels, companion cells, phloem fibers and phloem parenchyma.

(2) Structure of monotyledon roots (the cross section of stemona root)

Main points of observation on the ecto – entad structures are as follows:

① Velamen: It is the outer most row of slight polygon cells.

② Cortex

Ⅰ. Epicortex: It is composed by a layer of compact cells.

Ⅱ. Cortex: It is made up of many layers of small cells, the majority cells in root.

Ⅲ. Endodermis: It is the inner most layer of compact cells with Casparian dots.

③ Stele

Ⅰ. Pericycle: It is an enveloping cell in stele composed by 1 – 2 rows of small and tangential prolonging parenchyma cells, located below the endodermis.

Ⅱ. Xylem.

Ⅲ. Phleom.

(3) Secondary structure of dicotyledon roots (cross section of peony root)

Main points of observation on the ecto – entad structures are as follows:

① Periderm: It forms the secondary protective tissue with protecting function, made up of the cork layer, phellogen and phelloderm.

Ⅰ. Cork layer: Several orderly arranging layers of rectangle cork cells.

Ⅱ. Phellogen: It is formed by the pericyclic cells which resumed their fissionability again, situated under the cork layer.

Ⅲ. Phelloderm: It includes several layers of big parenchyma cells without chloroplast, the more developed phelloderm are also called secondary cortex.

② Vascular bundle: It is made up of phloem, cambium and xylem.

Ⅰ. Phloem: It includes the closely arranging cells outside the cambium and is made up of sieve tubes, companion cells, phloem parenchyma cells and phloem fibers. It is the conducting tissue, which transports organic nutrient substance produced by photosynthesis to the other parts of plant body.

Ⅱ. Cambium: It is the layer of closely arranging flat cells with fissionability, which forms secondary xylem inwards and secondary phloem outwards.

III. Xylem: It is inside the cambium and made up of radially arranging vessel dyed into red, wood fiber and wood parenchyma cells. Radially arranging wood rays are made up of 1 – 2 rows of parenchyma cells. Xylem, a kind of conducting tissue, transports water and soluble inorganic nutrient from lower to higher portions in plant body.

IV. Medullary rays: They are the radially arranging parenchyma cells between vascular bundles. Most of the dicotyledon roots don't possess pith.

(4) Anomalous structure of dicotyledon root (achyranthis radix)

Main points of observation on the ecto – entad structures are as follows:

① Periderm: It is made up of the cork layer, phellogen and phelloderm, but the phellogen and phelloderm are not easy to identify.

② Anomalous vascular bundle: The vessels with dyed red walls are the main part of xylem. Outside the xylem is phloem whose cells differ in size. These anomalous vascular bundles arrange in concentric rings.

③ Normal vascular bundle: It is diarch type situated in center.

4. The identification of powder of root type of crude drugs

Take the above materials powder, permeabilize with chloral hydrate and mount with dilute glycerol, observe the form of vessels, calcium oxalate crystals, phloem fibers, wood fibers and cork cells, etc.

Points in experiment report

1. Describe the morphologic characteristics of white peony root, red peony root, baical skullcap root and stemona root.

2. Draw the block – diagrams of cross section structures of wildginger, paeonia, achyranthis radix and stemona root. Sign the names of every tissue portion clearly.

3. Draw the microscopic characteristics pictures of powdered baical skullcap, white peony and balloon flower root and sign the names of every microscopic characteristic.

Topics for thinking

1. How many kinds of the familiar abnormal roots are present?

2. What are the main differences between the primary and secondary constructions of dicotyledon roots? How does the secondary construction form?

3. What are the similarities and differences between the primary constructions of dicotyledon and monocotyledon?

4. What is the abnormal root construction? How many kinds of the familiar abnormal roots are there?

5. What are the main differences between white peony and red peony root?

实验四 根类药材——人参、甘草、何首乌、麦冬的鉴定

【实验目的】

1. 掌握 人参（生晒参、红参、糖参）、甘草、何首乌、麦冬生药及饮片的性状鉴别特征；人参、甘草、何首乌、麦冬横切片的组织构造特征及粉末的显微鉴别特征。

2. 了解 人参、甘草、何首乌、麦冬药材的理化鉴别方法。

【实验材料】

1. **原植物的蜡叶标本** 人参、甘草、何首乌、麦冬。

2. **药材与饮片** 生晒参、红参、糖参、红参须、甘草、粉甘草、蜜炙甘草饮片、生首乌、制首乌、麦冬。

3. **石蜡横切片** 人参、何首乌、麦冬。

4. **粉末** 人参、甘草、何首乌、麦冬。

【实验仪器与试剂】

1. **仪器** 光学显微镜、载玻片、盖玻片、单面刀片、镊子、酒精灯、培养皿、纱布、小玻棒、擦镜纸、滤纸条、试管（10 ml）、小玻璃漏斗。

2. **试剂** 水合氯醛试液、稀甘油、蒸馏水、80% 浓硫酸、三氯化锑三氯甲烷饱和溶液、10% NaOH、HCl、氨试液、乙醚。

【实验内容】

一、原植物鉴定

观察人参、甘草、何首乌、麦冬原植物的形态特征。

二、性状鉴定

观察药材饮片的性状特征，比较其异同点。

观察要点：形态、药材表面、色泽、质地、气味、断面。

三、显微鉴定

1. **横切面观察** 分别取人参、甘草、何首乌、麦冬根横切片置于显微镜下，观察组织构造特征。

观察要点：木栓层、皮层、内皮层、异型维管束（云锦花纹）、树脂道、草酸钙晶体、韧皮部、形成层、木质部和维管束的特征，尤其注意单子叶植物麦冬的根毛、根被、黏液细胞及草酸钙针晶、分泌细胞、石细胞、内皮层、中柱鞘、韧皮部、木质部和髓（图 2-5、2-6、2-7）。

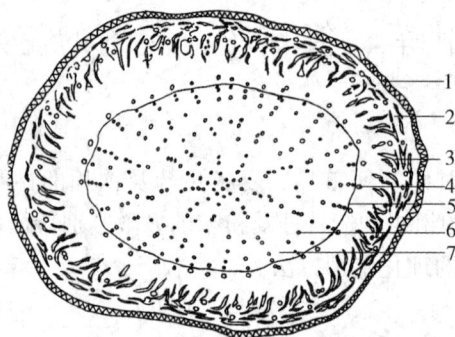

图 2-5 人参（根）横切面简图

1. 木栓层 2. 韧皮部 3. 裂隙
4. 树脂道 5. 形成层 6. 导管 7. 射线

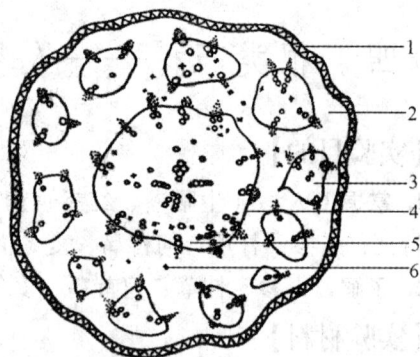

图 2-6 何首乌（块根）横切面简图

1. 木栓层 2. 皮层 3. 异型维管束
4. 形成层 5. 木质部 6. 簇晶

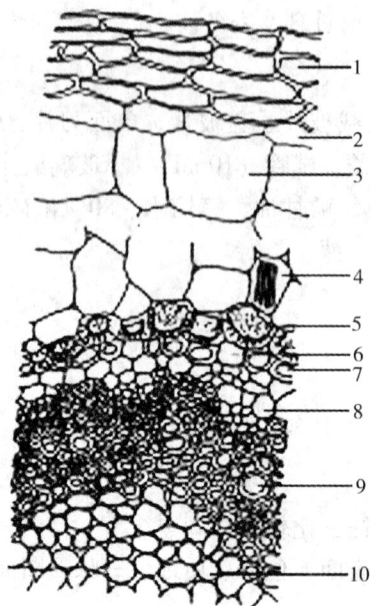

图 2-7 麦冬横切面

1. 根被 2. 外皮层 3. 皮层 4. 含晶黏液细胞
5. 石细胞 6. 通道细胞 7. 内皮层 8. 韧皮部
9. 木质部 10. 髓

2. 粉末观察 取人参、甘草、何首乌、麦冬粉末少许，用蒸馏水装片，镜检淀粉粒。用水合氯醛透化，稀甘油装片，观察草酸钙晶体、导管等组织构造特征。

观察要点：淀粉粒的形态、簇晶的大小及棱角的钝锐、晶纤维、方晶、木栓细胞的特点、导管的种类、树脂道、棕色细胞、黏液细胞、针晶、石细胞、通道细胞、柱晶的形态（图 2-8、2-9、2-10）。

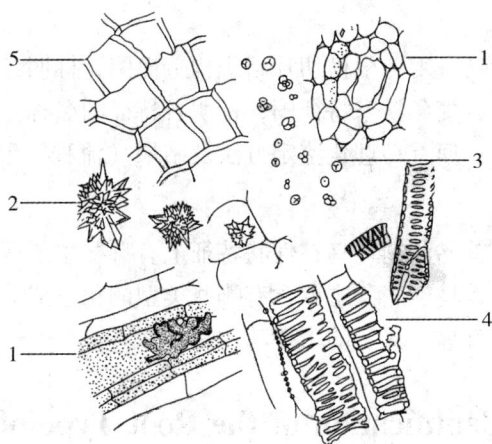

图 2-8　人参粉末显微特征图
1. 树脂道　2. 草酸钙簇晶　3. 淀粉粒
4. 导管　5. 木栓细胞

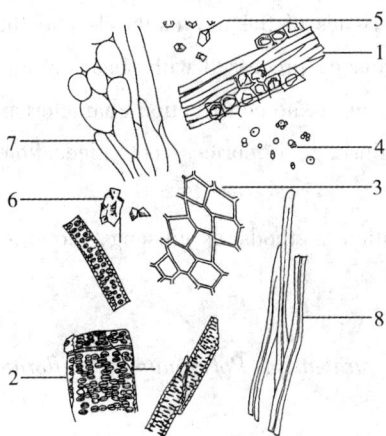

图 2-9　甘草粉末

1. 晶纤维　2. 导管　3. 木栓细胞　4. 淀粉粒
5. 草酸钙方晶　6. 棕色块　7. 射线细胞

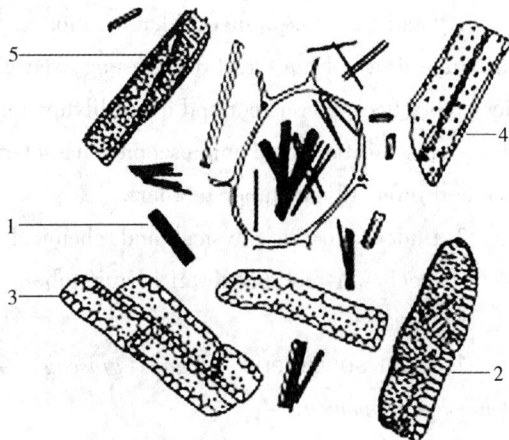

图 2-10　麦冬粉末

1. 草酸钙针晶及细柱状结晶　2. 石细胞
3. 内皮层细胞　4. 木纤维　5. 管胞

四、理化鉴别

1. 取人参粉末 0.5 g，加乙醇 5 ml，振摇，过滤，滤液少量置蒸发皿中蒸干，滴加三氯化锑三氯甲烷饱和溶液，蒸干显紫色（甾萜类）。

2. 取甘草粉末少许置白瓷板上，加 80%（V/V）硫酸数滴显黄色，渐变橙黄色（甘草甜素反应）。

3. 取生首乌粉末 0.1 g，加 10% 氢氧化钠溶液 10 ml，煮沸 3 分钟，冷后过滤。取滤液，加盐酸使成酸性，加等量乙醚振摇，醚层应显黄色。分取醚层 4 ml，加氨试液2 ml 振摇，氨液层显红色（蒽醌类反应）。

【报告要求】

1. 绘制人参、何首乌、麦冬根横切片组织构造简图，标明各组织构造名称。

2. 绘制人参、甘草、麦冬粉末特征图，标明各特征的名称。

3. 记录人参、甘草、何首乌理化鉴定方法及结果（流程图形式）。

【思考题】

1. 山参和园参、生首乌和制首乌在性状特征上有哪些主要区别点？

2. 人参、甘草、何首乌、麦冬主要含有哪些类型的化学成分？

3. 人参、甘草、何首乌、麦冬的主要功效是什么？

Experiment 4　Identification of the Root Type of Crude Drugs— Ginseng, Licorice Root, Fleeceflower Root and Dwarf Lilyturf Tuber

Aim

1. Learn the appearance, identification and characteristics of the raw materials and their cut crude drugs of ginseng (dry ginseng, red ginseng, ginseng processed with sugar), liquorices root, fleeceflower root and dwarf lilyturf tuber. Learn the tissue construction characteristics of the cross sections and microscopic characteristics of ginseng, liquorices root, fleeceflower root and dwarf lilyturf tuber powders.

2. Understand the physical and chemical identification methods of ginseng, liquorices root, fleeceflower root and dwarf lilyturf tuber.

Material

1. Plant specimens　*Panax ginseng*, *Glycyrrhiza uralensis*, *Polygonum multiflorum*, *Ophiopogon japonica*.

2. Crude drugs and cut crude drugs　Shengshaishen (dry ginseng), Hongshen (red ginseng), Tangshen (ginseng processed with sugar), Hongshenxu (red ginseng fibre), Gancao (liquorices root), Fengancao (unpeeled liquorices root), Mizhigancao (liquorices root processed with honey), Shengshouwu (fleeceflower root), Zhishouwu (processed fleeceflower root) and Maidong (dwarf lilyturf tuber).

3. Paraffin sections　Renshen (ginseng), Heshouwu (fleeceflower root) and Maidong (dwarf lilyturf tuber).

4. Powders　Renshen (ginseng), Gancao (liquorices root), Heshouwu (fleeceflower root) and Maidong (dwarf lilyturf tuber).

Equipment and reagents

1. Optical microscope, glass slide, cover glass, one side blade, nippers, alcohol lamp, culture capsule, gauze, glass stick, lens paper, filter paper, test tube (10 ml) and glass funnel.

2. Chloral hydrate solution, dilute glycerin, distilled water, 80% (*V/V*) sulfuric acid,

saturated chloroform solution of antimony trichloride, 10% sodium hydroxide, ethyl ether and ammonia solution.

Methods

1. Identification of Plant specimens

Observe the morphologic characteristics of *Panax ginseng*, *Glycyrrhiza uralensis*, *Polygonum multiflorum*, *Ophiopogon japonica*.

2. Appearance identification of crude drugs

Observe the morphologic characteristics of the crude drugs and their cut crude drugs and compare the similarity and difference.

Main points of observation: shape, color, texture, odor and cross – section.

3. Identification of microscopic characteristics

(1) Observation of the cross section slides   Test the cross section slides of ginseng, liquorices root, fleeceflower root and dwarf lilyturf tuber under microscope and observe their characteristics of tissue construction.

Main points of observation: cork layer, cortex, endodermis, anomalous vascular bundles (brocaded patterns), resin canals, calcium oxalate clusters, phloem, cambium, xylem and vascular bundles, especially pay attention to root hair, epidermis, mucous cells and raphides crystals, secretary cells, stone cells, endodermis, pericycle, phloem, xylem and pith of dwarf lilyturf tuber, a monocotyl plant.

(2) Observation of powder   take a bit of powder of crude drugs, mount with water and test their starch grains under microscope. Permeabilize with chloral hydrate, mount with dilute glycerin to observe the characteristics of calcium oxalate crystals, vessels, etc.

Main points of observation: the appearance of starch grains, the size and angularity of clusters, crystal fibers, square crystals, cork cells, varieties of vessels, appearance of resin canals, phloem parenchyma cells, mucous cells and raphides crystals, stone cells, passage cells and pillar crystals.

4. Physical and chemical identification

(1) Take 0.5 g of ginseng powder, add 5 ml of alcohol, shake, filter, evaporate a bit of the filtrate in an evaporating dish, add saturated antimony trichloride chloroform solution dropwise to dissolve the residue, evaporate to dryness and purple color appears (steroid and terpene) .

(2) Put a bit of liquorices root powder on white porcelain base plate, add 80% (*V/V*) sulfuric acid, yellow colour is shown and then change to orange yellow gradually (glycyrrhizin reaction) .

(3) Take 0.1 g of fleeceflower root powder, add 10 ml of 10% sodium hydroxide solution, boil for 3 min and filter it after cooled. Take the filtrate, acidify it with hydrochloric acid, shake after add the same amount of ethyl ether and the ether layer should show yellow. Take 4 ml ether solution, shake after add 2 ml of ammonia solution and the ammonia solution shows red (anthraquinone reaction) .

Points in experiment report

1. Draw the block diagram of the cross sections of ginseng, fleeceflower root and dwarf lilyturf tuber and sign the names of every portion clearly.

2. Draw the characteristics diagram of powder edginseng, liquorices root and dwarf lilyturf tuber and sign the names of every tissue structure clearly.

3. Record the physical and chemical identification methods and results of ginseng, liquorices root and fleeceflower root (in a fluidogram).

Topics for thinking

1. What are the main differences between wild ginseng and garden ginseng, fleeceflower root and its processed drugs?

2. What types of chemical compositions are contained in ginseng, liquorices root, fleeceflower root and dwarf lilyturf tuber?

3. What are the main effects of ginseng, liquorices root, fleeceflower root and dwarf lilyturf tuber?

实验五　茎、根茎类生药的组织构造

【实验目的】

1. 掌握　双子叶植物、单子叶植物地上茎的显微构造特征，比较其异同点。；蕨类植物根茎的初生构造、双子叶植物根茎的次生构造、异常构造的特点。

2. 识别　植物茎的性状特征，了解变态茎的形态特征及种类。

【实验材料】

1. 新鲜的植物体　紫丁香、天门冬、皂荚、丝瓜茎、玉竹、姜、唐菖蒲、百合、半夏。

2. 原植物蜡叶标本　金钗石斛、钩藤、大叶钩藤、薄荷、白木香、桑枝、桂枝、忍冬藤、桑寄生、首乌藤、通草、皂角刺、关木通、川木通、木通、粗茎鳞毛蕨、延胡索。

3. 生药和饮片标本　石斛、钩藤、沉香、桑枝、桂枝、忍冬藤、桑寄生、首乌藤、通草、皂角刺、关木通、木通、绵马贯众、延胡索。

4. 石蜡切片　石斛、沉香茎横切片；绵马贯众、石菖蒲、大黄根茎横切片。

【仪器与试剂】

1. 仪器　光学显微镜、载玻片、盖玻片、单面刀片、镊子、酒精灯、培养皿、纱布、小玻棒、擦镜纸、滤纸条、试管（10 ml）、小玻璃漏斗。

2. 试剂　水合氯醛试液、稀甘油、蒸馏水。

【实验内容】

一、观察植物

注意总结变态茎的类型。

二、观察各茎、根茎类药材的原植物蜡叶标本

注意关木通、川木通、木通叶的形态异同点；观察蕨类植物粗茎鳞毛蕨叶的形态、孢子囊群等特征。

三、观察各茎、根茎类的生药药材及饮片的性状特征

观察要点：注意观察各药材及饮片的形态、色泽、质地、断面、气味。比较关木通、川木通、木通的色泽、质地、断面等特征。

四、镜检石斛、沉香的石蜡切片

比较双子叶植物茎与单子叶植物茎在皮层、髓、维管束种类、维管束数目与排列方式等方面的区别。比较双子叶植物草质茎、木质茎的横切面显微组织构造的区别。

五、镜检绵马贯众根茎、石菖蒲根茎、大黄根茎横切片

观察要点：观察绵马贯众根茎横切片中分体中柱、细胞间隙腺毛、内皮层细胞、凯氏点等特征（图2-11）；石菖蒲根茎皮层中的纤维束、内皮层细胞的凯氏点、周木式维管束、油细胞及草酸钙方晶；大黄根茎横切面中异型维管束（星点）、导管、射线、维管束排列方式。

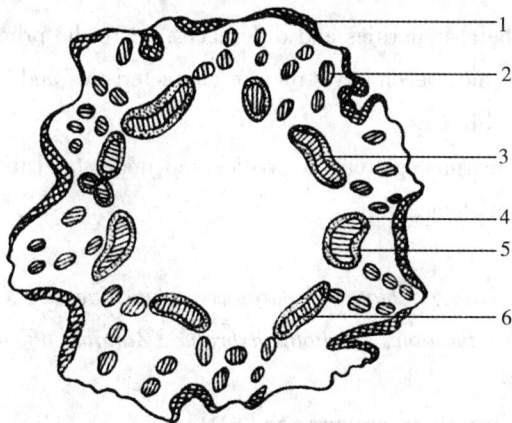

图2-11 绵马贯众根茎横切面简图
1. 厚壁组织 2. 叶迹维管束 3. 分体中柱
4. 内皮层 5. 韧皮部 6. 木质部

【报告要求】

1. 列表比较所观察的茎、根茎类药材主要的性状鉴别特征。

药材	形	色	表面	断面	质地	茎变态种类
钩藤						
沉香						
桑枝						
忍冬藤						
桑寄生						
延胡索						

2. 绘制石斛、沉香的横切面组织构造简图，标明各部位名称。

3. 绘制绵马贯众根茎、石菖蒲根茎组织构造简图，绘制大黄星点组织构造简图，标明各部位的名称。

【思考题】

1. 常见的变态茎有几种？

2. 根茎类生药与根类生药在组织构造方面有哪些主要区别点？蕨类植物、单子叶、双子叶植物根茎的组织构造有何异同点？

3. 何为根茎的异常构造？大黄的异常构造与何首乌的异常构造有何区别？

Experiment 5　The Tissue Structures of the Stem and Rhizome Types of Crude Drugs

Aim

1. Learn the microscopic structure characteristics of aerial stems of dicotyledon and monocotyledon and compare their similarities and differences. Learn the primary structure characteristics of pteridophyte rhizome, secondary structure characteristics and abnormal structure characteristics of dicotyledon rhizomes.

2. Identify the stem morphologic characteristics and understand the morphological characters and types of abnormal stems.

Material

1. Fresh Plants　*Syringa oblata*, *Asparagus cochinchinensis*, *Gleditsia sinensis*, *Luffa cylindlrica*, *Polygonatum odoratum*, *Gladiolus hybridus*, *Zingiber officimale*, *Lilium pumilum*, *Pinellia ternata*.

2. Original plant herbarium specimens　*Dendrobium nobile*, *Ramulus uncariae cum unci*, *Uncaria rhynchophylla*, *Mentha haplocalyx*, *Aquilaria sinensis*, *Ramulus mori*, *Caulis lonicerae*, *Taxillus chinensis*, *Caulis polygoni multiflori*, *Tetrapanax papyriferus*, *Spina gleditsiae*, *Caulis aristolochiae manshuriensis*, *Caulis clematidis armandii*, *Akebia quinata*, *Dryopteris crassirhizoma* and *Corydalis yanhusuo*.

3. Crude drugs and cut crude drugs　Shihu (dendrobium), Gouteng (rhynchophyl-

la), Chenxiang (Chinese eaglewood wood), Sangzhi (mulberry twig), Rendongteng (honey-suckle stem), Sangjisheng (mistletoe), Shouwuteng (tuber fleeceflower stem), Tongcao (medulla tetrapanacis), Guanmutong (manchurian aristolochia stem), Mutong (caulis hocquartiae), Mianmaguangzhong (basket fern rhizome) and Yanhusuo (corydalis tuber).

4. **Paraffin sections** Shihu (dendrobium), Chenxiangjing (Chinese eaglewood wood) (stem), Mianmaguanzhong (basket fern rhizome), Shichangpu (grassleaf sweetflag rhizome) and Dahuang (rhubarb).

Equipment and reagents

1. Optical microscope, slide, cover glass, blade, nippers, alcohol lamp, culture dish, gauze, glass stick, lens paper, filter paper, test tube (10 ml), glass funnel.

2. Chloral hydrate solution, dilute glycerine, distilled water.

Methods

1. Observe the fresh plants specimens and summarize the types of abnormal stems.

2. Observe the herbarium specimens of stem and rhizome types of crude drugs.

Pay attention to the similarities and differences of leaf properties between *Caulis aristolochiae manshuriensis and Caulis clematidis armandii and Akebia quinata*. Observe the leaf appearance of basket fern rhizome and the character of its sori.

3. Observe the morphologic characteristics of crude drug materials and cut crude drugs of stem and rhizome types of crude drugs.

Main points of observation: appearance, color, texture and odor; comparison of *Caulis aristolochiae manshuriensis, Caulis clematidis armandii* and *Akebia quinata*.

4. Test dendrobium and eaglewood paraffin sections under microscope.

Compare the dicotyledon and monocotyledon stem in aspect of cortex; pith; type, number and arrangement of vascular bundles. Compare microscopic tissue structure of their cross sections of dicotyledon herbaceous and woody stems.

5. Test the cross sections of basket fern rhizome stem, rhubarb and grassleaf sweetflag rhizome under microscope.

Main points of observation: meristele, intercellular glandular hair, endodermis cells and Casparian dots in basket fern rhizome section; fiber bundles, Casparian dots of endodermis cells, amphivasal bundles, oil cells and calcium oxalate square crystals in grassleaf sweetflag rhizome cortex; abnormal vascular bundles (asteria), vessels, rays, arrangement of vascular bundles on rhubarb cross section.

Points in experiment report

1. Compare the morphologic characteristics of stem or rhizome type of crude drugs in following table.

drug materials	property	color	surface	Cross section	texture	type of anomalous stem
rhynchophylla						
eaglewood						
mulberry twig						
honeysuckle stem						
Chinese taxillus herb						
corydalis tuber						

2. Draw the tissue structure diagram of the cross sections of dendrobium and eaglewood, and sign the names of each part.

3. Draw the tissue structure diagram of the cross sections of basket fern rhizome and grass-leaf sweetflag rhizome, star points of rhubarb and sign names of each portion.

Topics for thinking

1. How many types of common anomalous stems are present?

2. What are the main differences between the rhizome and root type of crude durgs? What are the similarities and differences of pteridophyte, monocotyledon and dicotyledon rhizomes?

3. What is the anomalous structure of rhizome? What are the differences of the anomalous structure between rhubarb and fleeceflower root?

实验六　根茎类药材——大黄、黄连、川芎、苍术的鉴定

【目的要求】

1. 掌握　双子叶植物根茎的组织构造特点；大黄、黄连、川芎、苍术粉末的显微鉴别特征；大黄、黄连的理化鉴定方法。

2. 了解　生药的显微化学定性分析及荧光分析方法。

【实验材料】

1. **原植物蜡叶标本**　掌叶大黄、唐古特大黄、药用大黄、虎杖、黄连、三角叶黄连、云南黄连、川芎、茅苍术、北苍术、白术、波叶大黄。

2. **生药和饮片标本**　大黄、波叶大黄、虎杖、味连、雅连、云连、川芎（纵切片）、苍术、白术。

3. **石蜡切片**　黄连（根茎）、川芎（根茎）、苍术（根茎）。

4. **药材粉末**　大黄、波叶大黄、黄连、川芎、苍术。

【实验仪器与试剂】

1. **仪器**　显微镜、临时装片用具、酒精灯、试管、回流装置、紫外分析仪、微量升华装置、恒温水浴锅。

2. **试剂**　水合氯醛试液、稀甘油、蒸馏水、浓盐酸、10%氢氧化钠溶液、NaHCO₃饱和溶液、乙醚、乙醇、1%香草醛的乙醇溶液、甲醇、稀盐酸、30%硝酸、硫酸、漂

白粉、5% 没食子酸乙醇溶液。

【实验内容】

一、观察各根茎类药材的原植物蜡叶标本

注意掌叶大黄、唐古特大黄及药用大黄叶的形态的异同点；注意观察伞形科植物川芎、菊科植物茅苍术的形态特征；注意黄连、三角叶黄连、云南黄连的形态异同点。

二、观察根茎类药材的生药及饮片的性状特征

观察要点：注意观察各药材及饮片的形态、色泽、质地、断面、划痕、气味。比较掌叶大黄、唐古特大黄、药用大黄的性状异同点；比较三种黄连的性状异同点；比较茅苍术、北苍术、白术的断面等特征。

三、镜检黄连根茎、苍术根茎、川芎根茎横切片

观察并比较它们组织构造特征的异同点。

观察要点：比较观察黄连根茎横切片中石细胞的分布与数目、韧皮纤维、根迹、叶迹维管束、髓等情况（图 2 - 12）；观察苍术根茎横切面中石细胞环带、大型油室、木纤维束、射线、薄壁细胞中的菊糖等情况；观察川芎根茎横切面中油室、木纤维、根迹维管束等情况（图 2 - 13）。

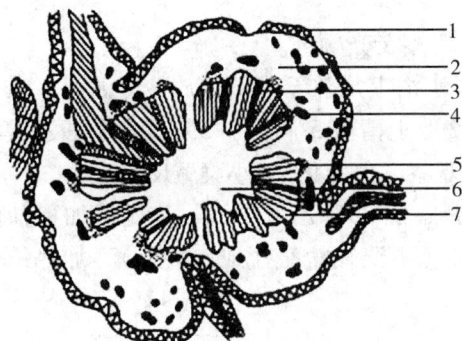

图 2 - 12　黄连根茎横切面简图
1. 木栓层　2. 皮层　3. 木化射线　4. 石细胞
5. 韧皮部　6. 髓　7. 木质部

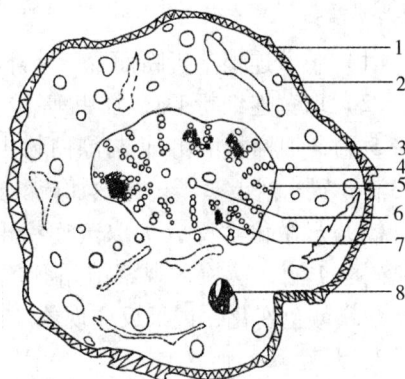

图 2 - 13　川芎横切面简图
1. 木栓层　2. 油室　3. 韧皮部　4. 形成层
5. 木质部　6. 髓　7. 木纤维　8. 根迹维管束

四、观察药材粉末

取大黄、黄连、川芎、苍术粉末少许，用水装片镜检，观察淀粉粒；用水合氯醛透化，稀甘油装片镜检，观察药材粉末的组织构造及后含物的显微鉴别特征。

观察要点：淀粉粒、草酸钙结晶（簇晶、针晶）、菊糖、纤维、木栓细胞等的形态，导管的种类（图 2 - 14、2 - 15）。

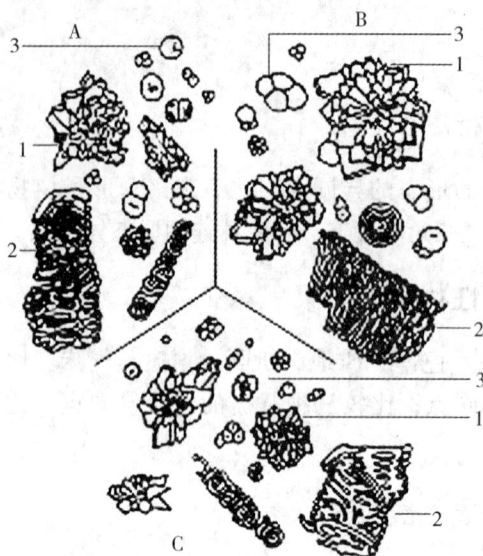

图 2-14 大黄粉末

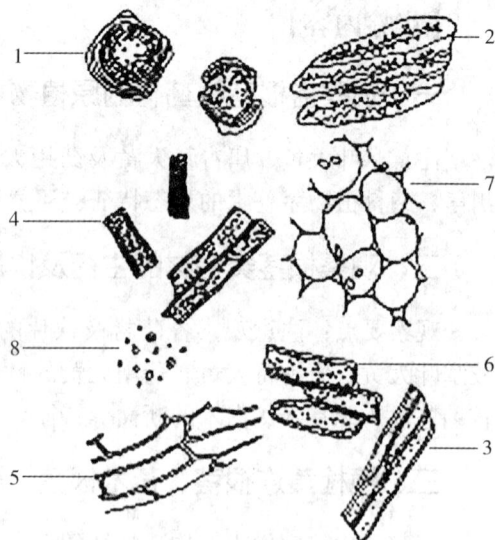

图 2-15 黄连粉末

A. 掌叶大黄 B. 药用大黄 C. 唐古特大黄

1. 草酸钙簇晶 2. 导管 3. 淀粉粒

1. 石细胞 2. 韧皮纤维 3. 木纤维 4. 导管 5. 鳞叶
表皮细胞 6. 木薄壁细胞 7. 草酸钙结晶 8. 淀粉粒

五、理化鉴别

1. 黄连

（1）将黄连根茎折断面置于紫外光下，观察荧光颜色。

（2）取黄连细粉 1 g，加甲醇 10 ml，置水浴上加热至沸腾，放冷，滤过。①取上清液 5 滴，加稀盐酸 1 ml 与漂白粉少量；②取上清液 5 滴，加 5% 没食子酸乙醇溶液 2~3 滴，置水浴上蒸干，趁热加硫酸数滴，观察颜色变化。（小檗碱反应）。

（3）显微化学反应　取黄连粉末或切片，加 70% 乙醇 1 滴，片刻后加稀盐酸或 30% 硝酸 1 滴，镜检，观察结晶颜色及形状（小檗碱盐酸盐或硝酸盐），加热结晶溶解，观察颜色变化，记录反应现象。

2. 大黄

（1）微量升华。取大黄粉末少许，置微量升华器中，盖上一载玻片，于石棉网上小火加热，使温度缓慢上升。待载玻片出现水汽或黄色升华物时，取下反转放冷，镜检升华物形状、颜色。从镜下取出载玻片，滴加 10% NaOH 1 滴，观察颜色变化。（羟基蒽醌类反应）

（2）取大黄及波叶大黄粉末或碎块少许，分别加稀醇溶液浸泡 10 分钟，不断振摇，放置后，分别吸取上清液约 0.5 ml 滴于滤纸上，置紫外灯下观察。比较二者荧光颜色。（检查土大黄苷）

（3）取大黄粉末 0.5 g，加 10% NaOH 溶液 10 ml，加热煮沸 5 分钟，放冷过滤，滤液以盐酸酸化（可从溶液颜色变化判定）。再加乙醚 5 ml 振摇，吸取上层醚液，加 NaHCO$_3$ 饱和溶液 2 ml。观察醚层、NaHCO$_3$ 液层的颜色，记录反应现象，并说明其原理。（大黄酸的鉴定反应）

【报告要求】

1. 绘制大黄、黄连、川芎、苍术粉末特征图，标明各组织构造名称。

2. 记录黄连理化鉴定方法及结果（流程图形式）。

3. 记录大黄理化鉴定方法及结果（流程图形式）。

4. 记录大黄酸鉴定反应方法及结果，并讨论原理。

【思考题】

1. 根茎类生药与根类生药在组织构造上有哪些主要区别点？

2. 大黄、黄连、川芎、苍术主要含有哪些类型的化学成分及具有哪些药理作用？

3. 大黄、黄连、川芎、苍术粉末分别具有哪些主要的组织构造特征？

Experiment 6 Identification of the Rhizome Type of Crude Drugs—Rhubarb, Coptis Root, Szechwan Lovage Rhizome and Atractylodes Rhizome

Aim

1. Learn the tissue construction characteristics of dicotyledon rhizome drugs. Learn the microscopic characteristics of powdered rhubarb, coptis root, Szechwan lovage rhizome and atractylodes rhizome. Learn the physical and chemical identification methods of rhubarb and coptis root.

2. Understand the methods of microscopic chemical qualitation reaction and fluorimetic analysis.

Material

1. Plant herbarium specimens *Rheum palmatum*, *Rheum tanguticum*, *Rheum officinale*, *Polygonum Cuspidati*, *Coptis chinensis*, *Coptis deltoides*, *Coptidis teetoides*, *Ligusticum chuanxiong*, *Atractylodes lancea*, *Atractylodes chinensis*, *Atrctylodis macrocephalae* and *Rheum undulatum*.

2. Crude drugs and proceeded drug specimens Dahuang (rhubarb), Boyedahuang (undulate rhubarb), Huzhang (giant knotweed rhizome), Yunlian (Coptis chinensis), Yalian (Coptis deltoids), Weilian (Coptidis teetoides), Chuanxiong (Szechwan lovage rhizome), Cangzhu (atractylodes rhizome) and Baizhu (largehead atractylodes rhizome).

3. Paraffin sections Huanglian (Coptis rhizome), Chuanxiong (Szechwan lovage rhizome) and Cangzhu (atractylodes rhizome)

4. Powders Dahuang (rhubarb), Boyedahuang (undulata rhubarb), Huanglian (Coptis rhizome), Chuanxiong (szechwan lovage rhizome) and Cangzhu (atractylodes rhizome).

Equipment and reagents

1. Microscope, temporary mounting appliance, alcohol lamp, test tube, refluxing installation, ultraviolet spectrophotometer, microsublimation installation and thermostatic waterbath.

2. Chloral hydrate solution, dilute glycerine, distilled water, concentrated hydrochloric

acid, 10% sodium hydrate solution, saturated sodium hydrocarbonate solution, ether, ethanol, methanol, dilute hydrochloric acid, 30% nitric acid, sulfuric acid, bleaching powder and gallic acid ethanol solution.

Methods

1. Observe plant herbarium specimens, pay attention to the similarities and differences of *Rheum palmatum*, *Rheum tanguticum* and *Rheum officinale*; pay attention to the morphologic characteristics of chuanxiong (*Umbelliferae*) and Cangzhu (*Compositae*) ; pay attention to the similarities and differences between three kinds of coptis rhizoma.

2. Observe the morphologic characteristics of crude drugs and cut crude drugs.

Main Points of observation: the form, color, texture, section, streak, odor. Compare the similarities and differences in morphologic characteristics between *Coptis chinensis*, *Coptis deltoides* and *Coptidis teetoides*; between *Rheum palmatum*, *Rheum tanguticum* and *Rheum officinale*; compare the section characteristics of Cangzu and Baizu.

3. Observe microscopic characteristics of cross sections of coptis, Cangzhu and Chuanxiong and compare the similarities and differences between their tissue construction characteristics.

Main Points of observation: distribution and number of stone cells, phloem fibers, root and leaf trace bundles and pith in golden thread rhizome section; anomalous bundles (asterion) , vessels, rays and arrangement vascular bundles on rhubarb rhizome section.

Observe the girdle bands in stone cells, large oil cavities, wood fiber bundles, rays, the inulin in parenchyma cells on atractylodes rhizome section; observe the oil cavities, xylons, root trace vascular bundles in Szechwan lovage rhizome.

4. Take a bit of powder of rhubarb, coptis rhizome, Szechwan lovage rhizome and atractylodes rhizome, mount with water and test starch grain under microscope. Permeabilize with chloral hydrate and mount with dilute glycerin to observe their microscopic characteristics of tissue structures and ergastic substances.

Main Points of observation: starch grains, calcium oxalate (cluster or raphides crystals) , inulin, fibers, cork cells and the varieties of vessels.

5. Physical and chemical identification.

(1) Coptis rhizoma

① Observe the fluorescence color of its rhizome section under ultraviolet light.

② Take 1 g of its fine powder, add 10 ml of methanol, heat until it is boiled in waterbath, cool and filter it.

Ⅰ. Take 5 drops of supernate liquid, add 1 ml dilute hydrochloric acid and a small quantity of bleaching powder and observe the color change.

Ⅱ. Take 5 drops of the supernate fluid, add 2 – 3 drops of 5% gallic acid ethanol solution, evaporate to dryness, add several drops of sulfuric acid when it is hot and observe the color change (2 reactions of berberine).

③ Microscopic chemistry reaction　Take some powder or a cross section, add 1 drop of

70% ethanol and 1 drop of dilute hydrochloric acid or 30% nitric acid and test the shape and color of the appeared crystals (muriate or nitrate of berberine) under microscope; heat to make the crystal dissolved, observe the change of color and record the reaction phenomenon.

(2) Rhubarb

① Microsublimation　Take a bit of powder, put into a microsublimating apparatus, cover with a glass slide, put them on asbestos gauze and heat with tiny fire to make the temperature rise gradually. When water vapor or yellow sublimate appears on the slide, change it; reverse the collected slide and cool, cover and test under microscope to observe the form and color of the sublimate. Then add 1 drop of 10% sodium hydroxide to the slide and observe the color change (reaction of hydroxyanthraquinones).

② Take a bit of powder or scrap of rhubarb and *Rheum frangenbachii*, soak with dilute alcoholic solution for 10 min respectively, shake continually, imbibe some of their supernate fluid with filter paper respectively, observe under ultraviolet lamp and compare their fluorescence color (inspecting of ponticin).

③ Bornträger reaction　Take 0.5 g of the rhubarb powder, add 10 ml of 10% sodium hydroxide solution, boil for 5 min, filter after cooling and acidify with hydrochloric acid (judge by the solution color change). Add 5 ml of ether, shake, imbibe the upper ether solution and add 2 ml of saturated sodium hydrocarbonate solution. Observe the color of the ether and sodium hydrocarbonate solution, record the phenomenon of reaction and explain the reaction principle (Identification of rhein).

Points in experiment report

1. Draw the microscopic characteristics of powdered rhubarb, coptis rhizome, Szechwan lovage rhizome and atractylodes rhizome amd indicate structures of each tissue clearly.

2. Take notes of the methods and results of the physical and chemical identification of coptis rhizome (in a fluidogram).

3. Take notes of the methods and results of the physical and chemical identification of rhubarb (in a fluidogram).

4. Take notes of the identification reaction of rhein and discuss its principle.

Topics for thinking

1. What are the main differences between rhizome and root types of crude drugs in aspect of tissue construction?

2. What types of chemical compounds are contained in rhubarb, coptis rhizome, Szechwan lovage rhizome and atractylodes rhizome and their pharmacological actions?

3. What are the obvious microscopic features of powdered rhubarb, coptis rhizome, Szechwan lovage rhizome and atractylodes rhizome?

实验七　根茎类药材—半夏、川贝母、天麻的鉴定

【目的要求】

1. 掌握　单子叶植物根茎的组织构造特点；天麻的理化鉴定方法；半夏、川贝母、

天麻粉末的显微鉴别特征。

2. 熟悉 单子叶植物根茎类生药的性状鉴别特点。

【实验材料】

1. **原植物蜡叶标本** 半夏、天南星、水半夏、石菖蒲、暗紫贝母、川贝母、甘肃贝母、梭砂贝母、浙贝母、天麻。

2. **生药和饮片标本** 天南星、半夏、水半夏、石菖蒲、松贝、青贝、炉贝、天麻。

3. **石蜡切片** 天麻（块茎）、半夏（块茎）横切片。

4. **药材粉末** 半夏、川贝母、浙贝母、天麻。

【实验仪器与试剂】

1. **仪器** 显微镜、临时装片用具、酒精灯、试管、回流装置、紫外分析仪、恒温水浴锅。

2. **试剂** 水合氯醛试液、稀甘油、蒸馏水、碘试液、乙醇。

【实验内容】

一、观察各根茎类药材的原植物蜡叶标本

注意暗紫贝母、川贝母、甘肃贝母、梭砂贝母的叶的形态异同点；注意观察天南星科植物半夏的叶脉、肉穗花序、佛焰苞等形态特征；观察兰科植物天麻的茎、叶、苞片、合蕊柱的特点。

二、观察根茎类药材及饮片的性状特征

观察要点：注意观察各药材及饮片的形态、色泽、质地、断面、划痕、气味。比较松贝、青贝、炉贝的性状（图2-16）；观察半夏的色泽、质地、断面、气味等特征。观察天麻块茎的性状特征（茎基、芽苞、圆脐形瘢痕、点状环纹、断面、质地等）。

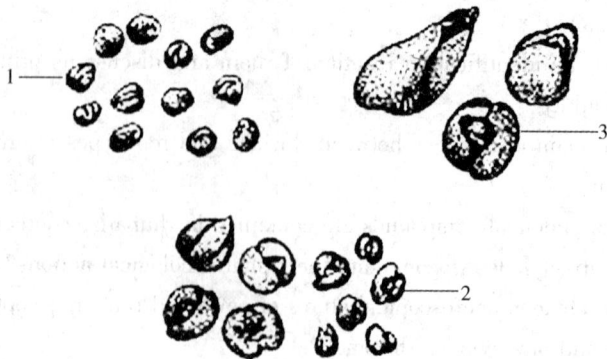

图2-16 川贝母药材
1. 松贝 2. 青贝 3. 炉贝

三、镜检天麻块茎、半夏块茎横切片

观察比较天麻块茎、半夏块茎组织构造特征的异同点。

观察要点：块茎横切面中维管束排列方式、多糖团块、草酸钙针晶束等情况。

四、观察药材粉末的组织构造及后含物的显微特征

取半夏、川贝母、浙贝母、天麻粉末少许，用水装片镜检，观察淀粉粒；用水合氯醛透化，稀甘油装片镜检，观察药材粉末的组织构造及后含物的显微鉴别特征。

观察要点：淀粉粒、多糖团块、草酸钙结晶（针晶、方晶）、厚壁细胞等的形态，气孔的类型，导管的种类（图 2 - 17、2 - 18、2 - 19）。

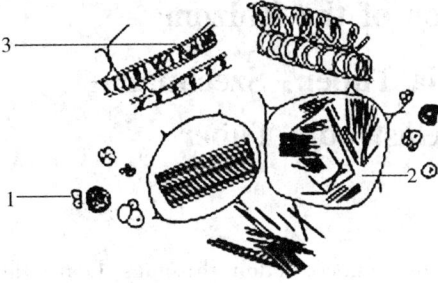

图 2 - 17　半夏粉末

1. 淀粉粒　2. 草酸钙针晶　3. 导管

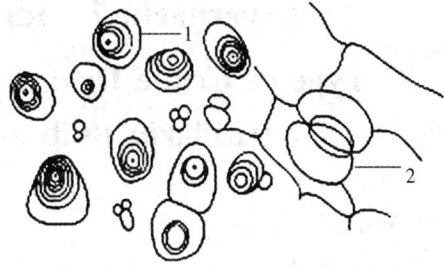

图 2 - 18　川贝母粉末

1. 淀粉粒　2. 气孔

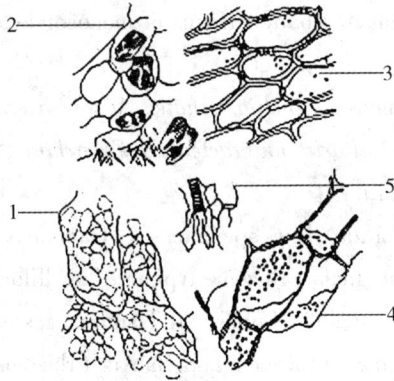

图 2 - 19　天麻粉末

1. 含糊化多糖类物质薄壁细胞（示颗粒）　2. 草酸钙针晶

3. 木化薄壁细胞　4. 薄壁细胞　5. 导管

五、天麻的理化鉴别

1. 粉末水提后加碘试液 2~4 滴，观察颜色变化。

2. 取粉末 0.2 g，加乙醇 10 ml，加热回流 1 小时，滤过，取滤液 1 ml 置 10 ml 量瓶中，加乙醇稀释至刻度，摇匀，以紫外分光光度计测定，在 270 nm ± 1 nm 波长处有最大吸收。

【报告要求】

1. 绘制天麻块茎横切面组织构造简图，标明各部位组织构造名称。

2. 绘制半夏、川贝母、天麻粉末特征图，标明各组织构造特征名称。

3. 记录天麻理化鉴定方法及结果。

【思考题】

1. 半夏、川贝母、天麻主要含有哪些类型的化学成分及主要药理作用？

2. 半夏、川贝母、天麻粉末鉴定主要具有哪些组织构造特征？

3. 归纳天麻的性状鉴别特征。

Experiment 7　Identification of the Rhizome Type of Crude Drugs — Pinellia Tuber, Szechuan – fritillaria Bulb and Tall Gastrodia Tuber

Aim

1. Learn the tissue construction characteristics of monocotyledon rhizomes. Learn the physical and chemical identification methods of tall gastrodia tuber. Learn the microscopic identification characteristics of pinellia tuber, szechuan – fritillaria bulb and tall gastrodia tuber.

2. Understand the morphologic characteristics of monocotyledon rhizome type of drugs.

Material

1. Plant herbarium specimens　*Pinellia ternate*, *Arisaema erubescens*, *Typhonium flagelliforme*, *Acorius tatarinowii*, *Fritillaria unibracteata*, *F. cirrhosa*, *F. przewalskii*, *F. delavayi*, *F. thunbergii* and *Gastrodia elata*.

2. Crude drugs and cut crude drug specimens　Tiannanxing (jackinthepulpit tuber), Banxia (pinelliae tuber), Shuibanxia (rhizome typhonii flagelliformis), Shichangpu (grassleaf sweetflag rhizome), Songbei, Qingbei, Lubei and Tianma (gastrodia rhizome).

3. Paraffin sections　Tianma (rhizome) and Banxia (rhizome).

4. Powders　Banxia, Chuanbeimu (szechuan – fritillary bulb), Zhebeimu (thunberg fritillary bulb) and Tianma.

Equipment and reagents

1. Microscope, temporary mounting appliance, alcohol lamp, test tube, refluxing installation, ultraviolet spectrophotometer and thermostatic waterbath.

2. Chloral hydrate solution, dilute glycerine, distilled water, iodine solution and ethanol.

Methods

1. Observe plant herbarium specimens, pay attention to the similarities and differences of leaves between all kinds of Fritillaria plants; pay attention to the characteristics of vein, spadix, spathe of pinelliae tuber (Araceae); observe the characteristics of stem, leaf, bract and gynostemium of tall gastrodia tuber (Orchidaceae).

2. Observe the morphologic characteristics of rhizomes and their cut crude drugs.

Main points of observation: form, color, texture, section, streak and odor. Compare the morphologic characteristics of color, texture, cross section and odor of three kinds of Szechuan – fritillaria bulb; observe the characteristics of color, texture, cross section and odor of pinelliae tuber. Observe the morphologic characteristics of tall gastrodia tuber (caudex, bud, umbiliform scar, punctiform rings, section and texture).

3. Microscopic characteristics of rhizome cross sections of tall gastrodia tuber and pinelliae tuber. Observe and compare the similarities and differences of their tissue construction.

Main points of observation: the arrangement of vascular bundles on the cross section, polysaccharides clumping and calcium oxalate raphides, etc.

4. Take a bit of powder of pinelliae tuber, szechuan – fritillary bulb, thunberg fritillary bulb and tall gastrodia tuber, mount with water and test starch grain under microscope. Permeabilize with chloral hydrate and mount with dilute glycerin to observe their characteristics of the tissue structures and ergastic substances.

Main points of observation: starch grains, polysaccharides clumping, calcium oxalate crystals (raphides, square crystals), sclerenchymatous cells, types of stoma and vessels.

5. The physical and chemical identification of tall gastrodia tuber

(1) Add 2 – 4 drops of iodine solution into the water extract of tall gastrodia tuber and observe the change of color.

(2) Take 0. 2 g of its powder, add 10 ml ethanol, heat and reflux for 1 hour, filter, take 1 ml of the filtrate to the volumetric flask (10 ml), dilute with ethanol to the scale, shake, determine with UV spectrophotometer and get the maximum absorption at the wave length of 270 nm ± 1 nm.

Points in experiment report

1. Draw the tissue structure diagrams of rhizome cross section of tall gastrodia tuber and indicate each part clearly.

2. Draw the powder characteristics picture of pinelliae tuber, Szechuan – fritillary bulb and tall gastrodia tuber and indicate each tissue structure clearly.

3. Take notes of the methods and results of the physical and chemical identification of tall gastrodia tuber.

Topics for thinking

1. What types of chemical compounds are contained in pinelliae tuber, Szechuan – fritillary bulb, tall gastrodia tuber and their pharmacological action?

2. What are the powder identification characteristics of pinelliae tuber, Szechuan – fritillary bulb and tall gastrodia tuber?

3. Sum up the morphologic characteristics of tall gastrodia tuber.

实验八　皮类药材——厚朴、黄柏、五加皮、肉桂、秦皮的鉴定

【实验目的】

1. 掌握　厚朴、黄柏、五加皮、肉桂粉末的显微鉴别特征；厚朴、黄柏、秦皮的理化鉴别方法。

2. 了解　皮类药材的性状鉴别特征。

【实验材料】

1. 原植物蜡叶标本　厚朴、凹叶厚朴、黄皮树、黄檗、肉桂、短梗五加、杜仲、秦皮、杠柳、牡丹。

2. 生药和饮片标本　厚朴（干皮、枝皮、根皮）、关黄柏、黄柏、肉桂、五加皮、杜仲、秦皮、香加皮、牡丹皮。

3. 石蜡切片　厚朴（干皮）、凹叶厚朴（干皮）、关黄柏、川黄柏。

4. 药材粉末　厚朴、黄柏、五加皮、肉桂、秦皮。

【实验仪器与试剂】

1. 仪器　光学显微镜、放大镜、载玻片、盖玻片、单面刀片、镊子、酒精灯、培养皿、纱布、小玻棒、擦镜纸、滤纸条、试管（10 ml）、小玻璃漏斗。

2. 试剂　水合氯醛试液、稀甘油、蒸馏水、三氯甲烷、乙醇、30% 硝酸、5% 三氯化铁的甲醇–水（1∶1）溶液、硝酸汞、间苯三酚。

【实验内容】

一、观察各皮类药材的原植物蜡叶

注意厚朴与凹叶厚朴、黄皮树与黄檗叶的形态异同点。

二、观察皮类药材的生药药材及饮片的性状特征

观察要点：注意观察各药材及饮片的形态，色泽、质地、断面、划痕、气味。比较厚朴的干皮、枝皮、根皮的油性的大小、断面等特征。比较关黄柏与川黄柏药材的性状。

三、镜检厚朴干皮、黄柏的石蜡切片

观察比较它们组织构造特征的异同点。

观察要点：注意观察厚朴干皮的栓内层石细胞环的分布、皮层中散在的纤维束、石细胞、油细胞的数目等特征。黄柏皮层中石细胞的分布与数目、韧皮纤维束切向排列层带的分布情况。

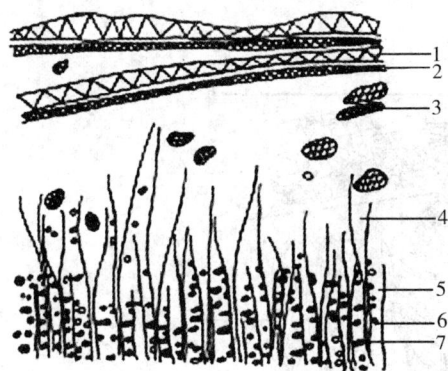

图 2 – 20　厚朴（树皮）横切面简图

1. 木栓层　2. 栓内层（石细胞层）　3. 石细胞群
4. 射线　5. 韧皮部　6. 油细胞　7. 纤维束

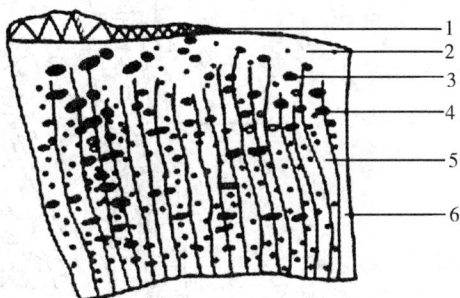

图 2 – 21　黄柏横切面简图

1. 木栓层　2. 皮层　3. 石细胞　4. 纤维
5. 韧皮纤维　6. 韧皮部

四、观察皮类药材粉末

取厚朴、关黄柏、五加皮、肉桂粉末少许，用水合氯醛透化，稀甘油装片镜检，观察药材粉末的组织构造及后含物的显微鉴别特征。

观察要点：草酸钙结晶、晶纤维、石细胞、油细胞、树脂道、纤维、筛管等的形态（图 2 – 22、2 – 23、2 – 24）。

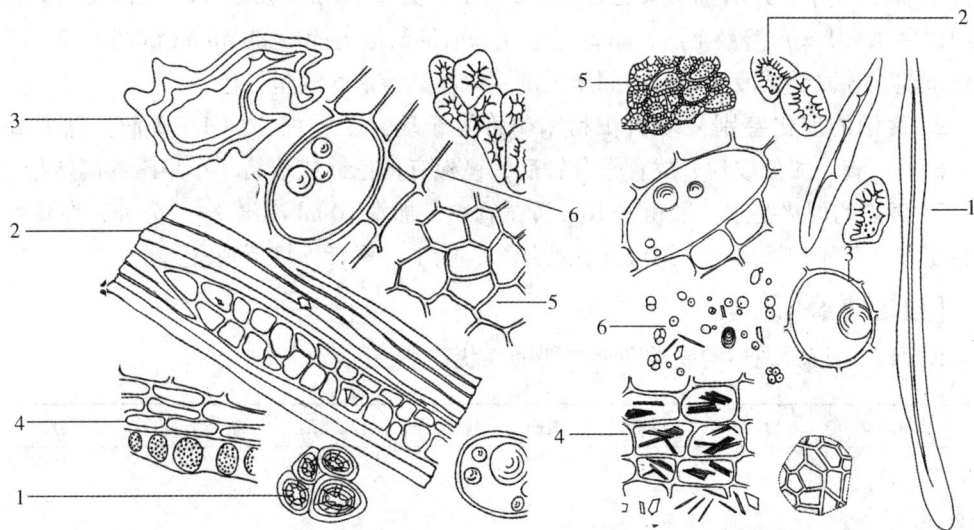

图 2 – 22　厚朴粉末

1. 石细胞　2. 射线细胞　3. 油细胞
4. 筛管分子　5. 木栓细胞
6. 草酸钙结晶

图 2 – 23　肉桂粉末

1. 纤维　2. 石细胞　3. 油细胞
4. 草酸钙针晶（射线细胞中）
5. 木栓细胞　6. 淀粉粒

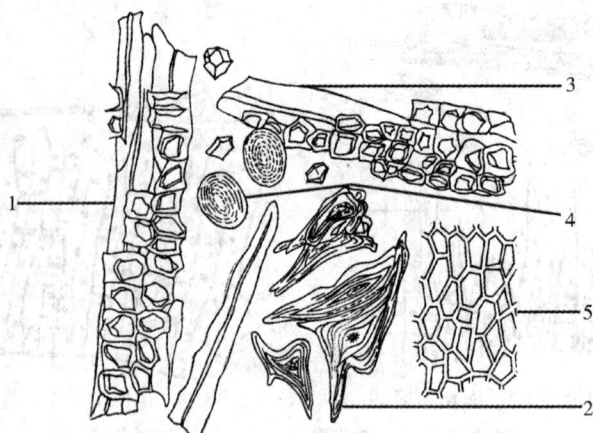

图 2 - 24 关黄柏粉末
1. 纤维及晶纤维
2. 石细胞 3. 草酸钙方晶
4. 黏液细胞 5. 木栓细胞

五、厚朴、黄柏、秦皮的理化鉴别

1. **厚朴的理化鉴别** 取厚朴粉末 3 g，用 30 ml 三氯甲烷提取，作为供试液。取供试液 15 ml，蒸干，残渣加 95% 乙醇 10 ml 溶解，滤过。①取滤液 1 ml，加 5% 三氯化铁的甲醇 – 水（1∶1）溶液 1 滴，呈蓝黑色；②取供试液 1 ml，加 Millon 试剂 1 滴，产生棕色沉淀；③取供试液 1 ml，加间苯三酚 – 浓盐酸溶液 5 滴呈红色。

2. **黄柏的理化鉴别** 取黄柏粉末少许置于玻片上，加乙醇 1 ~ 2 滴，然后滴加 30% 硝酸 1 滴，加盖玻片，放置数分钟后，镜检有黄色针状结晶（小檗碱的硝酸盐）。

3. **秦皮的理化鉴别** 取粉末 10 g 置试管中，加水 10 ml 冷浸 3 ~ 5 分钟，在日光下观察是否有荧光，然后将水溶液滴在滤纸上，吹干，置紫外灯下观察荧光。

【报告要求】

1. 列表比较所观察的皮类药材主要的性状鉴别特征。

药材	形	色	表面	断面	质地	断面结晶	荧光
关黄柏							
黄柏							
牡丹皮							
厚朴							
肉桂							
杜仲							
秦皮							

2. 绘制关黄柏与厚朴横切片组织构造简图，标明各部位名称。

3. 绘制厚朴、黄柏、五加皮、肉桂粉末特征图，标明各组织构造、细胞后含物名称。

4. 记录厚朴、黄柏、秦皮的理化鉴定方法及结果（流程图形式）。

【思考题】

1. 皮类生药横切片组织构造有哪些主要特点？

2. 厚朴、黄柏、秦皮的主要化学成分及药理作用有哪些？

3. 厚朴、黄柏、五加皮、肉桂主要具有哪些粉末鉴定特征？

Experiment 8　Identification of the Bark Type of Crude Drugs — Magnolia，Phellodendron，Acanthopanax，Cinnamon and Ash Barks

Aim

1. Learn the microscopic characteristics of powdered magnolia, phellodendron, acanthopanax and cinnamon barks. Learn the physical and chemical identification methods of magnolia, phellodendron and ash barks.

2. Understand the morphologic characteristics of the bark type of crude drugs.

Material

1. Plant herbarium specimens　*Magnolia officinalis*，*Magnolia officinalis* var. *biloba*，*Phellodendron chinense*，*Phellodendron amurense*，*Cinnamomum cassia*，*Acanthopanax sessifloru*，*Eucommiae ulmoides*，*Fraxinus rhynchophylla*，*F. chinensis*，*F. chinensis* var. *acuminata*，*F. stylosa*，*Periploca sepium* and *Paeonia suffruticosa*.

2. Crude drugsand their cut crude drug specimens　Houpo（magnolia bark，trunk bark，shoot bark，root bark），Guanhuangbai（amurense corktree bark），Huangbai（chinense corktree bark），Rougui（cinnamon bark），Wujiapi（acanthopanax bark），Duzhong（eucommia bark），Qinpi（ash bark），Xiangjiapi（Chinese sikvine root bark）and Mudanpi（moutan cortex）

3. Paraffin sections　magnolia bark（trunk bark），biloba magnolia bark（trunk bark），Guanhuangbai and Chuanhuangbai.

4. Powders　Houpo, Guanhuangbai, Wujiapi, Rougui and Qinpi.

Equipment and reagents

1. Optical microscope, magnifying glass, glass slide, cover glass, single plane blade, nippers, alcohol lamp, culture capsule, absorbent gauze, glass stick, lens paper, filter – paper, sample tube and glass funnel.

2. Chloral hydrate solution, dilute glycerine, distilled water, chloroform, ethanol, 30% nitric acid, methanol water（1∶1）solution of 5% chloride ferric, mercuric nitrate and 1，3，5 – trihydroxybenzene hydrochloric acid solution.

Methods

1. Observe plant herbarium specimens, pay attention to the similarity and difference of the

leaf form between *Magnolia officinalis* and *Magnolia officinalis* var. *biloba*; between *Phellodendron chinense* and *Phellodendron amurense*.

2. Observe the morphologic characteristics of bark drugs and their cut crude drugs.

Main points of observation: form, color, texture, section, streak and odor. Compare the characters of oiliness and cross sections of magnolia trunk, shoot and root bark. Compare the morphologic characteristics of *Phellodendron amurense* and *Phellodendron chinense*.

3. Test cross sections of magnolia trunk bark and phellodendron bark under microscope, observe and compare the similarity and difference of their tissue construction.

Main points of observation: the distribution of stone cell rings in phelloderm, the number of fiber bundles, stone cells and oil cells scattered in the cortex of magnolia bark; the distribution and number of stone cells in the cortex, the tangential zone distribution of phloem fiber bundles in phellodendron bark.

4. Take a bit of magnolia, phellodendron, acanthopanax and cinnamon barks powder, permeabilize with chloral hydrate and mount with dilute glycerin to observe their characters of tissue structures and ergastic substances.

Main points of observation: the form of calcium oxalate crystals, crystal fibers, stone cells, oil cells, resin canals, fibers, sieve tubes and the varieties of vessel.

5. The physical and chemical identification of magnolia, phellodendron and ash barks.

(1) The physical and chemical identification of magnolia bark   Take 3 g of magnolia bark powder, extract with 30 ml chloroform as the sample solution for test. Take 15 ml of the test solution, evaporate to dryness, dissolve the residue with 95% alcohol and filter. ① take 1 ml of the solution; add 1 drop of methanol water solution (1:1) of 5% chloride ferric and blue – black color appears. ② take 1 ml of the solution and add one drop of mercuric nitrate solution and brown sediment appears. ③ take 1 ml of the solution, add 5 drops of 1, 3, 5 – trihydroxybenzene hydrochloric acid solution and red color appears.

(2) The physical and chemical identification of phellodendron bark   Take a bit of phellodendron bark powder ona piece of slide, add 1 –2 drops of ethanol and 1 drop of 30% nitric acid solution, cover with a coverslip, put aside for several minutes and test appeared yellow needle crystals under microscope (berberine nitrate).

(3) The physical and chemical identification of ash bark   Put 10 g of ash bark powder into a test tube, sodden with 10 ml of cold water for 3 – 5 min and observe if the solution shows the fluorescence under the sunlight; then drop the water solution on filter paper, blow to dryness and observe its fluorescence under an ultraviolet lamp.

Points in experiment report

1. Compare the main morphological characters of the observed bark type of drugs in following table.

Drugs	Form	Color	Surface	Cross section	Texture	Crystal in cross section	Fluorescence
Phellodendron amurense							
Phellodendronchinense							
Paeonia suffruticosa							
magnolia bark							
cinnamon bark							
eucommia bark							
ash bark							

2. Draw the tissue diagrams of cross sections of phellodendron and magnolia barks, and indicate each part clearly.

3. Draw the powder characters of magnolia, phellodendron, acanthopanax and cinnamon barks, and indicate the names of each tissue structure and ergastic substances.

4. Take notes of the methods and results of physical and chemical identificationof magnolia, phellodendron and ash barks.

Topics for thinking

1. What are the main tissue construction characteristics of the bark type of crude drugs?

2. What kinds of constituents are contained in magnolia, phellodendron, ash barks and what are their pharmacological actions?

3. What are the powder microscopic characteristics of magnolia, phellodendron, acanthopanax and cinnamon barks?

实验九 叶类、全草类生药——麻黄、薄荷、大青叶、洋地黄叶、颠茄叶的鉴定

【实验目的】

1. 掌握 叶类、全草类生药的组织构造及显微特征；叶类、全草类生药的理化鉴别特征。

2. 了解 叶类、全草类生药的形态特征。

【实验材料】

1. **原植物蜡叶标本** 草麻黄、细辛、薄荷、石斛、广藿香、淫羊藿、益母草、石韦、穿心莲、车前草、绞股蓝、青蒿、菘蓝、洋地黄、颠茄、番泻、侧柏叶、艾叶。

2. **生药和饮片标本** 麻黄、细辛、薄荷、石斛、广藿香、淫羊藿、益母草、石韦、穿心莲、车前草、绞股蓝、青蒿、大青叶、银杏叶、洋地黄叶、颠茄叶、番泻叶、毛花洋地黄叶。

3. **石蜡切片** 草麻黄茎、薄荷茎、薄荷叶、颠茄叶。

4. **生药粉末** 麻黄、大青叶、薄荷、洋地黄叶。

【实验仪器与试剂】

1. **仪器** 显微镜、载玻片、盖玻片、酒精灯、纱布、小玻棒、擦镜纸、吸水纸、微量升华器、电炉、试管。

2. **试剂** 水合氯醛、稀甘油、蒸馏水，0.5%盐酸，碘化铋钾试液，碘化汞钾试液，10%氢氧化钠试液，乙醚，10%硫酸铜试液，浓硫酸，香草醛结晶、乙醇、氨试液、三氯甲烷、发烟硝酸、氢氧化钾试液、固体氢氧化钾、碱式醋酸铅试液、冰醋酸、三氯化铁试液、Kedde试液。

【实验内容】

一、观察叶类、全草类生药的原植物蜡叶标本

观察要点：植物形态，各器官特征。

二、观察叶类、全草类生药

观察要点：注意观察各药材及饮片的形态、色泽、质地、断面、气味。

三、镜检麻黄茎、薄荷茎、薄荷叶、颠茄叶石蜡切片

观察麻黄茎横切片的两棱线间下陷的气孔、下皮纤维束、皮层散在的纤维束、中柱鞘纤维束、外韧式维管束、髓及草酸钙方晶或砂晶（图2-25）。

观察薄荷茎横切片的表皮、皮层、维管束、髓（图2-26）。比较双子叶植物茎与单子叶植物茎在皮层、髓、维管束种类、维管束数目与排列方式等方面的区别。比较双子叶植物草质茎、木质茎的横切面显微组织构造的区别。

观察叶类药材横切面中腺毛、非腺毛、栅栏组织、海绵组织、维管束排列方式、叶肉细胞中结晶形状、颜色、厚角组织等（图2-27、2-28）。

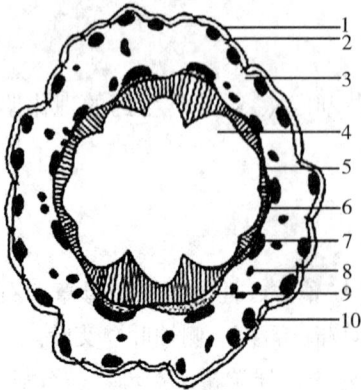

图2-25 草麻黄（茎）横切面

1. 表皮 2. 气孔 3. 皮层 4. 髓部
5. 形成层 6. 木质部 7. 中柱鞘纤维
8. 皮层纤维 9. 韧皮部 10. 下皮纤维

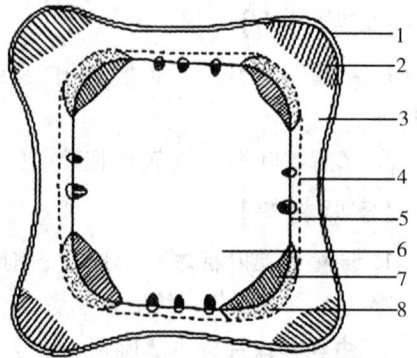

图2-26 薄荷（茎）的横切面

1. 表皮 2. 厚角组织 3. 皮层
4. 内皮层 5. 形成层 6. 髓
7. 木质部 8. 韧皮部

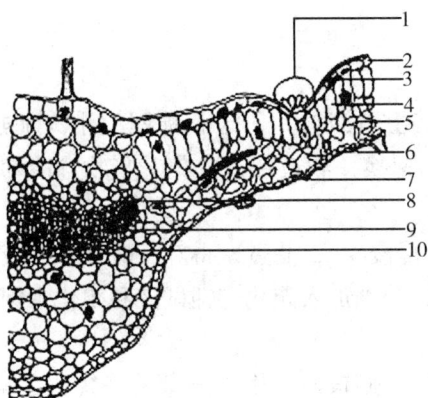

图 2-27　薄荷（叶）横切面

1. 腺鳞　2. 上表皮　3. 橙皮苷结晶

4. 栅栏组织　5. 海绵组织　6. 下表皮

7. 气孔　8. 厚角组织　9. 木质部

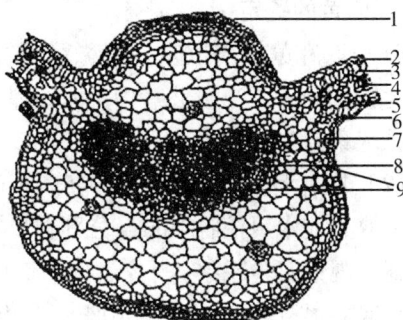

图 2-28　颠茄（叶）横切面

1. 厚角组织　2. 上表皮　3. 栅栏组织

4. 砂晶细胞　5. 海绵组织　6. 气孔

7. 下表皮　8. 木质部　9. 韧皮部

四、镜检麻黄、大青叶、洋地黄叶粉末的观察

取麻黄、大青叶、颠茄叶粉末少许，用水合氯醛透化，稀甘油装片镜检，观察药材粉末的组织构造及后含物的显微鉴别特征。

观察要点：麻黄的气孔侧面观保卫细胞呈哑铃形或电话筒形（图 2-29）；大青叶的靛蓝结晶、不等式气孔；薄荷叶的腺鳞及橙皮苷结晶、直轴式气孔、腺毛、非腺毛；洋地黄叶的不定式气孔，及它们的腺毛、非腺毛、表皮细胞、厚壁细胞的形态，气孔、导管的类型等。

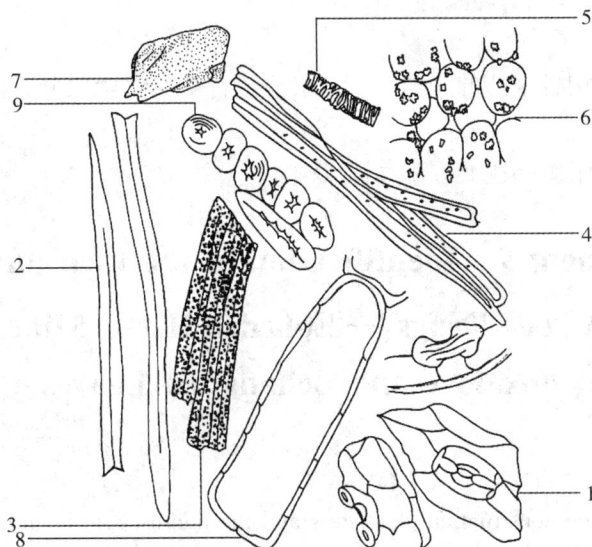

图 2-29　草麻黄（茎）粉末

1. 气孔　2. 皮部纤维　3. 嵌晶纤维（示草酸钙砂晶）　4. 木纤维

5. 导管　6. 皮层薄壁细胞　7. 色素块　8. 髓部薄壁细胞　9. 石细胞

五、理化鉴定

1. 麻黄的鉴定

（1）取麻黄粉末适量，置微量升华器中，盖上一载玻片，于石棉网上小火加热，使温度缓慢升高。当载玻片内的水汽消失时，迅速换一载玻片，收集升华物，冷却后镜检，观察升华物形态。

（2）取麻黄粉末 10 g，加 0.5% 盐酸 80 ml，冷浸 4 h，滤过，得麻黄酸性水浸液。

①取上述水浸液各 1 ml，分别置 2 支试管中，分别加入碘化铋钾试液和碘化汞钾试液 1 滴，观察实验现象。

②取酸水浸液 2 ml，用 10% 氢氧化钠试液调至强碱性，用乙醚萃取，挥去乙醚，残渣用盐酸溶液 2 ml 溶解，加 10% 硫酸铜试液 1 滴后，再加 10% 氢氧化钠溶液至显紫色，再加乙醚数毫升振摇后放置，观察醚层及水层颜色。

2. 薄荷的鉴定　取薄荷粉末适量，进行微量升华，所得油状物略放置，镜检，观察实验现象；加浓硫酸 2 滴及香草醛结晶少量，观察颜色变化，再加蒸馏水 1 滴，观察溶液颜色。

3. 洋地黄叶的理化鉴别　Kedde 反应：洋地黄叶甲醇提取液，滴于滤纸上，再滴加 Kedde 试液（3，5 - 二硝基苯甲酸 1 g 溶于 50 ml 甲醇，加 1 mol/L KOH 50 ml）少许，记录反应结果。（检查五元不饱和内酯环）

【报告要求】

1. 绘制草麻黄茎、薄荷茎、薄荷叶横切片的组织构造简图。
2. 绘制麻黄、大青叶、洋地黄叶的粉末组织构造图。
3. 记录麻黄、薄荷、洋地黄叶理化鉴定过程及结果，对实验现象进行讨论。

【思考题】

1. 本实验中所用各生药的来源、产地、显微特征、化学成分、药理作用及主要功效是什么？
2. 叶类生药在组织构造上有哪些特点？

Experiment 9　Identification of the Leaf and Herb Types of Crude Drugs — Ephedra Herb, Mint, Indigowood, Foxglove and Belladonna Leaves

Aim

1. Learn the tissue construction characters and the microscopic identification characters of leaf and herb types of crude drugs. Learn physical and chemical identification methods of leaf and herb types of crude drugs.

2. Understarnd the morphologic identification of leaf and herb types of crude drugs.

Materials

1. Plant herbarium specimens   *Ephedra sinica*, *Asarum heterotropoides*, *Mentha haplocalyx*, *Dendrobium nobile*, *Agastache rugosus*, *Epimedium brevicornum*, *Leonurus heterophyllus*, *Pyrrosia sheareri*, *Andrographis paniculata*, *Artemisia annua*, *Isatis indigotica*, *Digitalis purpurea*, *Atropa belladonna*, *Cassia angustifolia*, *Platycladus orientalis* and *Eriobotrya japonica*

2. Crude drugs and theircut crude drugs   Mahuang (ephedra herb), Xixin (wildginger), Bohe (mint), Shihu (caulis dendrobii), Guanghuoxiang (cablin patchouli herb), Yinyanghuo (epimedium herb), Yimucao (motherwort), Shiwei (pyrrosia leaf), Chuanxinlian (kalmegh), Cheqiancao (plantain), Jiaogulan (gynostemma), Qinghao (sweet wormwood herb), Daqingye (Indigowoad Leaf), Yinxingye (ginkgo leaf), Yangdihuangye (foxglove leaf), Dianqieye (belladonna leaf), Fanxieye (senna leaf) and Maohuayangdihuangye (grecian foxglove leaf).

3. Paraffin sections   Caomahuang (stem), Bohe (stem and leaf) and Dianqieye (leaf)

4. Powders   Caomahuang, Daqingye, Bohe and Yangdihuangye.

Equipment and reagents

1. Microscope, glass slide, cover glass, alcohol lamp, absorbent gauze, glass stick, lens paper, absorbent – paper, microsublimation installation, electric stove and test tube.

2. Chloral hydrate, dilute glycerine, distilled water, 0.5% hydrochloric acid, Potassium Heptaiodobismuthate solution, potassium mercuric iodide solution, 10% sodium hydroxide, diethyl ether, 10% copper sulfate solution, concentrated sulfuric acid, vanillin, ethanol, ammonia solution, chloroform, fuming nitric acid, potassium hydroxide solution, solid potassium hydroxide, lead subacetate solution, glacial acetic acid, ferric chloride solution and Kedde solution.

Methods

1. Observe plant herbaria of each leaf and herb types of drug materials above, pay attention to their appearance and characteristics of every organ.

2. Observe the morphological characters of leaf and herb types of crude drugs and their cut crude drugs.

Main points of observation: form, color, texture, section and odor.

3. Test the paraffin sections of ephedra herb, mint stem, mint leaves and belladonna leaves under microscope.

On cross – sections of ephedra herb, observe the cryptopole between two ridges, hypodermal fiber bundles, scattering fiber bundles in the cortex, collateral bundles, pith and square and sand crystals of calcium oxalate.

On cross – section of mint stem, observe epidermis, cortex, vascular bundle and pith. Compare dicotyledon and monocotyledon stem stem in the cortex and pith, the type of vascular bundle, the difference between the vascular bundle number and arrangement, etc. Comparison of the microstructure difference between herb stem, woody stem of dicotyledonous plants.

On cross – sections of leaf type of drugs, observe the glandular hair, glandular scales, nonglandular hair, palisade tissue, spongy tissue, arranging style of vascular bundles; crystal form, color and collenchyma in diachyma cells.

4. Test the powder of ephedra herb, indigowoad and foxglove leaves under microscope.

Take a bit of ephedra herb, indigowoad and foxglove leaves powder, permeabilize with chloral hydrate, mount with dilute glycerine and observe the tissue construction characters and ergastic substances.

Main points of observation: the lateral view of stoma shows dumbbell or telephone form (ephedra herb); indigo blue crystals and anisocytic type stomas (indigowoad leaf); glandular hair, nonglandular hair, glandular scales, aurantiamarin crystals and diacytic type stomas (mint leaf); anomocytic type of stomas (foxglove leaf); and their glandular hair, nonglandular hair, epidermic cells, sclerenchymatous cells and types of vessels.

5. The physical and chemical identification of ephedra herbs, mint and digitalis leaf.

(1) Identification of ephedra herbs

① Take a bit of powder, put into a microsublimation apparatus, cover with a slide, and heat on a slight fire to make temperature heighten gradually. When the water vapor on the slide disappears, change a slide quickly, gather the sublimate, cool and test the sublimate appearance under microscope.

② Take 10 g of powder; add 80 ml of 0.5% hydrochloric acid, sodden with cold water for 4 hours and filtrate to get the acidic infusion.

I. Take 1 ml of the infusion separately, put into two test tubes, add 1 drop of potassium heptaiodobismuthate solution and potassium mercuric iodide solution, respectively and observe the experiment phenomenon.

II. Take 2 ml of the infusion, adjust with 10% sodium hydroxide solution to strong alky, extract with diethyl ether, evaporate the diethyl ether, dissolve the residue with 2 ml of hydrochloric acid, add one drop of 10% copper sulfate solution and some drop 10% sodium hydroxide solution and purple color appears; add several drops of diethyl ether, shake, put aside and observe the color of the ester and water layer.

(2) Identification of mint Take some powder, microsublimate, obtain some oily liquid, put aside, test under microscope and observe the experiment phenomenon; add two drops of concentrated sulfuric acid and a bit of vanillin crystals and observe the change of color; add one drop of distilled water and observe color of the solution.

(3) Identification of foxglove leaf Kedde reaction: drop its methanol extraction solution on a filter paper, add a bit of Kedde test solution (dissolve 1 g of 3, 5 – dinitrobenzoic acid into 50 ml of methanol and add 50 ml of 1 mol/L KOH), and record the reaction result. (Examining the unsaturated five – carbon lactone ring)

Points in experiment report

1. Draw the detailed tissue diagrams of stem cross sections of ephedra herbs and mint.

2. Draw the microscopic characters disgrams of ephedra herb, indigowoad and foxglove leaves powder.

3. Record the procedure and results of the physical and chemical identification of ephedra herb, mint and foxglove leaf.

Topics for thinking

1. What are theoriginal plants, habitats, microscopic characteristics, chemical compositions, pharmacological actions and main effects of the crude drugs in this experiment?

2. What are the tissue construction characteristics of leaves?

实验十　花、果实、种子类生药的鉴定

【实验目的】

掌握　花、果实、种子类生药的原植物形态特征及药材性状；花、种子的结构和果实的分类；花、果实、种子类生药的显微鉴别特征；花、果实、种子类生药的理化鉴定方法。

【实验材料】

1. **原植物蜡叶标本**　辛夷、洋金花、金银花、红花、菊花。

2. **新鲜的花**　若干种。

3. **生药和饮片标本**　洋金花、金银花、红花、番红花、菊花、小茴香、北五味子、补骨脂、吴茱萸、山茱萸、陈皮、枸杞、山楂、乌梅、金樱子、连翘、马钱子、苦杏仁、桃仁、酸枣仁、牵牛子、砂仁、胖大海、槟榔、决明子、天仙子、白扁豆。

4. **石蜡切片**　小茴香、马钱子表皮毛茸。

5. **药材粉末**　洋金花、红花、金银花、北五味子、苦杏仁、马钱子。

【实验仪器与试剂】

1. **仪器**　显微镜、放大镜、临时装片用具。

2. **试剂**　水合氯醛、稀甘油、蒸馏水、10%碳酸钠、醋酸、乙醇、1%硫酸溶液、氨试液、三氯甲烷、发烟硝酸、氢氧化钾、三硝基苯酚试纸。

【实验内容】

一、观察各花、果实、种子类药材的原植物蜡叶标本

注意观察用药部位的形态特征。

二、观察新鲜的花

解剖新鲜的花，除观察花萼、花冠、雄蕊、雌蕊、柱头、子房、苞片外，用刀片切开子房，观察心皮包围而成的室及室内的胚珠。

三、观察各类药材的性状特征

注意观察各花类药材的形态，色泽、质地、气味。重点比较红花、番红花的性状特征的不同。

（1）观察果实类生药饮片，了解果实的形态特征，熟悉果实的分类。

观察要点：果实的形状、大小、颜色、顶端、基部、表面、质地、破断面、气味等。

（2）观察种子类生药饮片，了解种子的形态特征。

观察要点：种子的形状、大小、颜色、表面纹理、种脐、合点和种脊的位置、质地、气味等。

四、观察洋金花、红花、金银花粉末

取洋金花、红花、金银花粉末少许，用水合氯醛透化，稀甘油装片镜检，观察药材粉末的组织构造及后含物的显微鉴别特征。

观察要点：花粉粒、萌发孔、腺毛、非腺毛、草酸钙砂晶、方晶、簇晶、花冠表皮细胞、花柱碎片、分泌细胞、气孔的类型、导管等（图 2－30、2－31、2－32）。

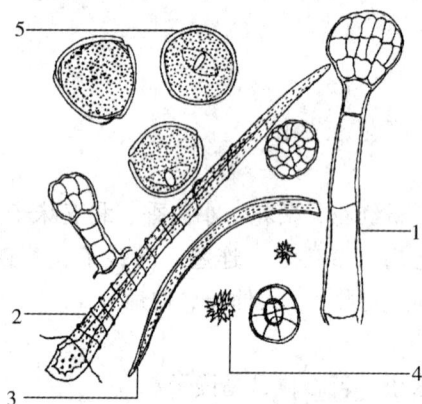

图 2－30　金银花粉末

1. 腺毛　2. 厚壁非腺毛　3. 薄壁非腺毛

4. 草酸钙砂晶　5. 花粉粒

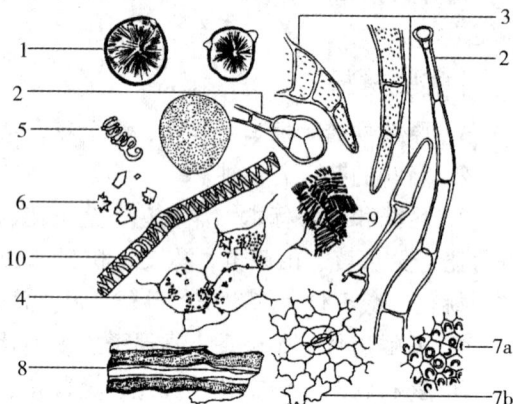

图 2－31　洋金花粉末

1. 花粉粒　2. 腺毛　3. 非腺毛　4. 草酸钙砂晶

5. 草酸钙方晶　6. 草酸钙簇晶　7. 花冠表皮

8. 黄棕色团块　9. 花粉囊内壁细胞　10. 导管

五、果实的内部构造观察

取小茴香的石蜡切片，置显微镜下观察其组织构造。

观察要点：中果皮有 6 个油管，接合面有 2 个，背面每二棱线间各有 1 个；棱线处有维管束柱；种脊维管束；内胚乳细胞含细小草酸钙簇晶（图 2－33）。

六、种皮构造的观察

取马钱子表皮毛茸的切片，观察其形态特征。

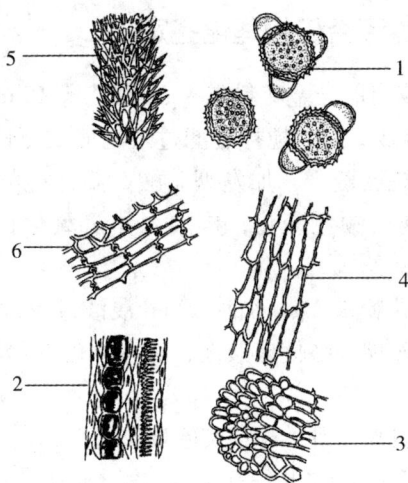

图 2 - 32　红花粉末

1. 花粉粒　2. 分泌管碎片　3. 花瓣顶端细胞

4. 花瓣细胞　5. 柱头细胞　6. 花药中部细胞

观察特点：毛茸单细胞，壁强木化，极厚，顶端钝圆，基部似石细胞状、内胚乳细胞壁厚，细胞呈细波状弯曲（图 2 - 34）。

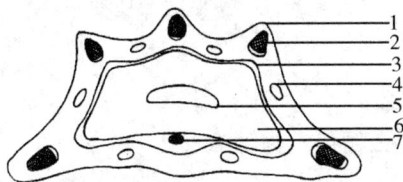

图 2 - 33　小茴香分果横切面

1. 外果皮　2. 维管束柱　3. 内果皮　4. 油管

5. 胚　6. 内胚乳　7. 种脊维管束

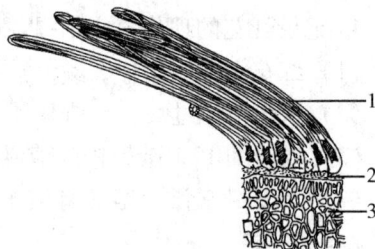

图 2 - 34　马钱子表皮毛茸

1. 表皮　2. 颓废的种皮细胞　3. 胚乳

七、观察北五味子粉末

取北五味子粉末少许，用水合氯醛透化装片，置显微镜下观察。

观察要点：果皮表皮细胞表面有微细角质线纹，可见类圆形或多角形油细胞，其周围有 6 ~ 7 个细胞围绕、种皮外表皮右细胞多角形，壁厚、种皮内层石细胞壁厚，纹孔较大而密。

八、观察苦杏仁粉末

取苦杏仁粉末少许，用水合氯醛透化装片，置显微镜下观察。

观察要点：种皮石细胞侧面观呈贝壳形，正面观呈类圆形或类多角形、种皮外表皮薄壁细胞多皱缩与石细胞相连、子叶细胞含细小草酸钙簇晶。

九、洋金花、红花、苦杏仁的理化鉴定

1. **洋金花的 Vitali 反应** 取洋金花粉末 4 g，加乙醇 15 ml，振摇约 15 分钟，滤过。滤液蒸干后，加 1% 硫酸溶液 2 ml，搅拌后滤过。滤液加氨试液呈碱性，用三氯甲烷 2 ml 振摇、提取，取三氯甲烷层蒸干，加发烟硝酸 5 滴，再蒸干，残渣冷却后加入氢氧化钾乙醇试液 2 ~ 3 滴，观察颜色变化，再加固体氢氧化钾一小块，记录反应结果。（莨菪烷类生物碱）

2. **红花的鉴定** 取红花粉末 2 g，加水 20 ml 浸渍过夜，过滤；残渣加 10% 碳酸钠溶液 8 ml 浸渍，滤过，滤液加醋酸使成酸性，观察颜色变化，记录反应结果。

3. **苦杏仁的鉴定**

（1）取苦杏仁数粒，加水共研，观察实验现象。

（2）取苦杏仁数粒，捣碎，称取约 0.1 g，置试管中，加 1% 稀硫酸数滴使湿润，试管中悬挂 1 条三硝基苯酚试纸，滴加 10% 碳酸钠溶液数滴湿润试纸，用软木塞塞紧，置热水浴中加热 10 分钟，观察试纸颜色。

【报告要求】

1. 绘金银花、红花、北五味子和苦杏仁的粉末特征图，标明各显微特征名称。

2. 绘小茴香、马钱子的横切面简图。

3. 记录洋金花的 Vitali 反应、苦杏仁的苦味酸钠反应的现象及结果。

4. 记录红花的理化鉴定结果并回答下列问题：

（1）红花水浸液显什么颜色？为什么？

（2）水溶液滤过后，残渣显什么颜色？为什么？

（3）残渣加 10% 碳酸钠溶液浸渍，滤液显什么颜色？为什么？

（4）加 10% 碳酸钠溶液有何作用？

【思考题】

1. 花类生药在组织构造上有哪些特点？果实、种子类生药的主要显微特征是什么？

2. 各类果实的性状特征是什么？

3. 洋金花、红花、番红花、北五味子、苦杏仁、马钱子主要化学成分及药理作用？

4. 列表比较红花、番红花的异同点。

Experiment 10   Identification of the Flower, Fruit and Seed Types of Crude Drugs

Aim

Learn the morphologic characteristics of the flower, fruit and seed types of crude drugs. Learn the structures of flower and seed, and classification of fruit. Learn the microscopic identification characteristics of the flower, fruit and seed types of crude drugs. Learn the physical and chemical identification methods of the flower, fruit and seed types of crude drugs.

Material

1. Plant herbarium specimens　*Magnolia biondii*, *Datura metel*, *Lonicera japonica*, *Carthamus tinctorius* and *Chrysanthemum morifolium*.

2. Fresh flowers　Several kinds.

3. Crude drugs and their cut crude drugs specimens　Yangjinhua (datura flower), Jinyinhua (honeysuckle flower), Honghua (safflower), Fanhonghua (saffron), Juhua (chrysanthemum), Xiaohuixiang (cumin), Beiwuweizi (Chinese magnoliavine fruit), Buguzi (psoralea fruits), Wuzhuyu (evodiae fructus), Shanzhuyu (cornel), Chenpi (orange peel), Gouqi (medlar), Shanzha (hawthorn fruit), Wumei (smoked plum), Jinyingzi (chrokee rose fruit), Lianqiao (forsythia suspensa), Maqianzi (curare), Kuxingren (bitter apricot seed), Taoren (peach seed), Suanzaoren (jujube seed), Qianniuzi (kaladana), Sharen (villous amomum fruit), Pangdahai (boat – fruited sterculia), Binlang (areca seed), Juemingzi (cassiac torae semen), Tianxianzi (henbane) and Baibiandou (lablab semen).

4. Paraffin sections　Xiaohuixiang and epidermis hair of Maqianzi.

5. Powders　Yangjinhua, Honghua, Jinyinhua, Beiwuweizi, Kuxingren and Maqianzi.

Equipment and reagents

1. Microscope, magnifying glass and temporary mounting appliance.

2. Chloral hydrate, dilute glycerine, distilled water, 10% natrium carbonicum, acetic acid, ethanol, 1% sulfuric acid solution, ammonia solution, chloroform, fuming nitric acid and potassium hydroxide solution, 2, 4, 6 – trinitrophenol test paper.

Methods

1. Observe each plant herbarium specimen and pay attention to the morphologic characteristics of the parts used for medicines.

2. Dissect fresh flowers to observe calyx, corolla, stamen, pistil, stigma, ovary and bract; cut ovary and observe the locule (including ovule) surrounded by carpels.

3. Observation of the morphologic characteristics of the flower types crude drugs.

Main points of observation: form, color, texture and odor. Pay attention to compare the morphologic characteristics difference between safflower and saffron.

(1) Observe the fruit type of crude drugs and their cut crude drugs and understand their morphologic characteristics and types of fruits.

Main points of observation: form, size, color, apex, basis, surface, texture, cross section, odor, etc.

(2) Observe seed type of crude drugs and their cut crude drugs and understand the morphologic characteristics of seeds.

Main points of observation: form, size, color, surface texture, hilum, the positions of chalaza and raphe, texture and odor.

4. Take a bit of datura flower, safflower and honeysuckle flower powder, permeabilize with chloral hydrate and mount with dilute glycerin to observe their characters of tissue structures

and ergastic substances.

Main points of observation: pollen grains, germinal apertures, glandular hair, nonglandular hair, calcium oxalate sand crystals, square crystals, druse crystals, corolla epidermic cells, style fragments, secretary cells, types of stomas, vessels, etc.

5. Take the paraffin section of cumin and observe its tissue structures under microscope.

Main points of observation: six vittaes inmesocarp, two on commissural surface and one between every two ridges on back side; vascular bundles on ridges; raphe vascular bundles and calcium oxalate druses in endosperm cells.

6. Observation of the tissue structures of episperm.

Take the paraffin section of epidermal hair of curare and observe its microscopic characteristics.

Main points of observation: unicellular hair with lignified and thickened cell walls, the circular apex and stone cell like base; endosperm cells with thickened walls and their intercellular spaces show sinuose.

7. Take a bit of Chinese magnoliavine fruit powder, permeabilize with chloral hydrate and observe under microscope.

Main points of observation: there are fine horny streaks on the surface of carpodermis epidermic cells; round or polygon oil cells surrounding by 6 – 7 cells can be seen all around; testa exocuticle cells with thickened cell walls are polygon form; testa stone cells possess large and dense pits and thickened cell walls.

8. Take a bit of bitter apricot seed powder, permeabilize with chloral hydrate, mount with dilute glycerin and observe under microscope.

Main points of observation: the testa stone cells shows shell – shaped in lateral view, show round or polygon in anterior view; testa exocuticle parenchyma cells mostly shrink and connect to stone cells; cotyledon cells possess tiny calcium oxalate druse crystals.

9. The physical and chemical identification of datura flower, safflower and bitter apricot seed.

(1) Vitali reaction ofdatura flower　Add 15 ml of ethanol into 4 g of datura flower powder and shake for about 15 min and filter. Evaporate to dryness, then add 2 ml of 1% sulfuric acid, churn and filter, basify the filtrate with ammonia solution, add 2 ml of chloroform and shake, evaporate the chloroform layer to dryness and add 5 drops of fuming nitric acid into the residue, evaporate again and cool the residue, add 2 – 3 drops of ethanol solution of potassium hydroxide, observe the change of color; add a bit of solid potassium hydroxide and record the reaction results (for tropane alkaloid).

(2) Add 20 ml of water into 2 g of safflower powder and soak overnight, filtrate andmacerate the residue with 8 ml of 10% sodium carbonate solution, filtrate again and acidify the filtrate with acetate acid, observe the change of color and record the result of reaction.

(3) Identification of bitter apricot sead

Ⅰ. Take several pills of bitter apricot seed, grind with water and observe the experiment phenomenon.

Ⅱ. Take several pills of bitter apricot seed, pound into pieces, weigh about 0. 1 g and put into a test tube. Dabble by drops of 1% sulfuric acid solution, hang a piece of 2, 4, 6 – trinitrophenol test paper moistened with 10% sodium carbonate solution in the test tube stoppered with a cork, heat in a warm bath for 10 min and observe the test paper color.

Points in experiment report

1. Draw the microscopic characters diagram of datura flower, safflower, Chinese magnoliavine fruit and bitter apricot seed powder and indicate each tissue structure clearly.

2. Draw the block diagram of cross – section structures of fennel and curare.

3. Take notes of the phenomenon and results of Vitali reaction of datura flower and Trinitrophenol reaction of bitter apricot seed.

4. Record the results of the physical and chemical identification of safflower, and answer the following questions:

(1) What is the water extraction color of safflower? Why?

(2) After filtrate, what is the color of residue left? Why?

(3) After the residue is soaked by 10% sodium carbonate and is filtered, what color will the filtrate show? Why?

(4) What is the purpose of adding 10% natrium carbonate solution?

Topics for thinking

1. What are the main tissue construction characteristics of the flower type of crude drugs? What are the main microscopic characteristics of the fruit and seed types of crude drugs?

2. What are the morphologic characteristics of each kind of fruit?

3. What kinds of chemical compounds are contained in datura flower, safflower, saffron, Chinese magnoliavine fruit, bitter apricot seed and curare, and what are their pharmacological actions?

4. Compare the similarities and differences between safflower and saffron.

实验十一 动物类生药——鹿茸的鉴定

【实验目的】

掌握 鹿茸药材的性状鉴别方法；生药鹿茸的理化鉴别特征。

【实验材料】

鹿茸药材、鹿茸对照药材、甘氨酸对照品。

【实验仪器与试剂】

1. **仪器** 光学显微镜、具塞锥形瓶、量筒、漏斗、滤纸、层析缸、硅胶 G 预制板、载玻片、盖玻片。

2. 试剂 稀甘油、蒸馏水、正丁醇、冰醋酸、乙醇、茚三酮、丙酮。

【实验内容】

一、基源动物鉴定

观察梅花鹿、马鹿的形态特征。

二、鹿茸药材性状鉴定

观察生药鹿茸药材花鹿茸和马鹿茸的性状。

观察要点：大小、形状、分支、外皮、颜色、锯口、气味。

三、显微鉴别

观察要点：表皮角质层，毛茸，骨碎片，未骨化骨组织，角化梭形细胞。

四、理化鉴别

取本品粉末 0.4 g，加 70% 乙醇 5 ml，超声处理 15 分钟，滤过，取滤液作为供试品溶液。另取鹿茸对照药材 0.4 g，同法制成对照药材溶液，再取甘氨酸对照品，加 70% 乙醇制成每 1 ml 含 2 mg 的溶液，作为对照品溶液，吸取供试品溶液和对照药材溶液各 8 μl、对照溶液 1 μl，分别点于同一硅胶 G 薄层板上，以正丁醇 – 冰醋酸 – 水（3 : 1 : 1）为展开剂，展开，取出，晾干，喷以 2% 茚三酮丙酮溶液，在 105℃ 加热至斑点显色清晰。供试品色谱中，在与对照药材色谱及对照品相应位置上，显相同颜色的斑点。

【报告要求】

1. 记录鹿茸药材的性状特征。
2. 记述显微鉴别方法及结果。
3. 记述理化鉴别方法及结果。

【思考题】

1. 生药鹿茸的基源动物是什么？伪品有哪些？如何区分？
2. 花鹿茸和马鹿茸在形状上有何异同点？
3. 鹿茸主要含有哪些类型的化学成分？这些化合物主要有哪些药理作用或功效？

Experiment 11　Identification of Animal Crude Drug—Pilose Antler

Aim

Learn the morphologic characteristics of pilose antler. Learn the physical and chemical identification methods of pilose antler.

Material

Medical material of pilose antler, reference drug of pilose antler, standard article of glycine.

Equipment and reagents

1. Optical microscope, conical flask with block, graduated cylinder, funnel, filter paper, laminar analysis chute, prepared thin layer plate, glass slide, cover glass.

2. Dilute glycerine, distilled water, n – butanol, glacial acetic acid, ethanol, ninhydrin, acetone.

Methods

1. Observe the appearance of origin animal.

2. Morphological identification.

Observe the morphous of *Cervus nippon* and *C. elaphus*.

Main points of observation: size, shape, branches, outer fur, color, cutting section and odor.

3. Microscopic identification.

Main points of observation: cutin layer of epidermit, hair, bone fragment, uncalcification bone tissue, cutin – like spindle cell.

4. Physical and chemical identification.

To 0. 4 g of the powder add 5 ml 70% ethanol, ultrasonicate for 15 minutes, filter, and use the filtrate as the test solution. Prepare a solution of 0. 4 g of Cornu Cervi Pantotrichum reference drug in the same manner as the reference drug solution. Dissolve glycine CRS in 70% ethanol toobtain the 2 mg/ml reference solution. Carry out the method for thin layer chromatography, usint silica gel G mixed with carboxymethylcellulose sodium as the coating substance and a mixture of n – butanol, glacial acetic acid and water (3 : 1 : 1) as the mobile phase. Apply separately to plate 8 μl of the test solution and the reference drug solution respectively, and 1 μl of the reference solution. After developing and removal of the plate, dry in the air. Spray with 2% solution of ninhydrin in acetone and heat at 105 ℃ to the spots clear. The main spots in the chromatogram obtained with the test solution correspond in position and colour to the spots in chromatogram obtained with the reference drug solution. The spot in the chromatogram obtained with the test solution corresponds in position and colour to the spot in the chromatogram obtained with the reference solution.

Points in experiment report

1. Record the morphologic characteristics of pilose antler.

2. Record the results of microscopic identification.

3. Describe the methods and results of the physical and chemical identification.

Topics for thinking

1. What are the original animals of pilose antler? And what are the fake articles? How to distinguish them?

2. What are the differences between Hualurong and Malurong?

3. What are the main components in pilose antler? And what kind of pharmacological func-

tions or Chinese function for them?

实验十二 动物类生药——蟾酥的鉴定

【实验目的】

1. 掌握 蟾酥药材的性状鉴别特征；蟾酥药材的理化鉴定方法；高效液相色谱仪的构造及使用方法；蟾酥药材的含量测定方法。

【实验材料】

1. 动物标本 中华大蟾蜍和黑眶蟾蜍动物标本。

2. 药材 蟾酥生药材及粉末。

3. 对照品 脂蟾毒配基对照品，华蟾酥毒基对照品。

【仪器与试剂】

1. 仪器 岛津 10Avp 型高效液相色谱仪，UV 检测器，ODS C – 18 反相色谱柱（150 mm × 4.6 mm，5 μm），微量进样器（25 μl），一次性滤器（0.45 μm），超声波仪，薄层板（5 cm × 28 cm）一块，乳钵，大层析缸，牛角勺，紫外灯，10 ml、20 ml 和 100 ml 量筒和 50 ml 具塞锥形瓶各一个，玻棒，25 ml 锥形瓶 2 个，10 ml、25 ml 和 100 ml 量瓶各一个，中直径 10 cm 蒸发皿 1 个，100 ml 小烧杯 2 个，玻璃滴管，小漏斗，10 ml 试管，毛细管，脱脂棉，滤纸，大头针，载波片，盖玻片。

2. 试剂 甲醇，乙醇，乙腈（色谱纯），重蒸水，磷酸二氢钾，稀甘油，蒸馏水，浓硫酸，稀碘液，二甲氨基苯甲醛固体，三氯甲烷，二氯甲烷，醋酐，硅胶 G，苯，丙酮，1% CMC – Na 溶液。

【实验内容】

一、基源动物鉴定

观察中华大蟾蜍、黑眶蟾蜍的形态特征。

二、性状鉴定

观察团酥、片酥商品药材的性状。

观察要点：注意药材的外形、颜色、质地、断面、气味等性状特征。

三、显微鉴定

取蟾酥粉末少许，进行下列显微鉴定。

（1）稀甘油装片镜检，呈半透明不规则碎块，并附有沙粒状固体。

（2）浓硫酸装片镜检，显橙黄色或橙红色，碎块四周逐渐缩小而成透明的类圆形小块，表面显龟裂纹理，放置稍久逐渐溶解消失。

（3）蒸馏水装片，加碘试液观察，不应显蓝色（检查淀粉）。

四、理化鉴定

1. 吲哚类生物碱反应　取蟾酥粉末约 0.1 g 置于 25 ml 锥形瓶中，加甲醇 5 ml 超声波提取 5 分钟后滤过，滤液置于 10 ml 试管中，加二甲氨基苯甲醛固体少许，滴加浓硫酸数滴，显蓝紫色。

2. 甾体类化合物反应　取蟾酥粉末约 0.1 g 置于 25 ml 锥形瓶中，加二氯甲烷 5 ml 超声波提取 5 分钟后滤过，将滤液置于蒸发皿中蒸干，残渣用 1 ml 醋酐溶解，转移至 10 ml 试管中，沿管壁缓缓滴加浓硫酸，初显蓝紫色，渐变蓝绿色。

3. 紫外鉴定　取蟾酥粉末约 0.1 g 置于 25 ml 锥形瓶中，加二氯甲烷 10 ml 超声波提取 10 分钟后滤过，将滤液置于蒸发皿中蒸干，残渣用 5 ml 乙醇溶解作为供试液。取脂蟾毒配基对照品 1 mg，加乙醇 5 ml 制成对照品溶液。取供试液和对照品溶液分别测定紫外吸收光谱，于波长 220～400 nm 处进行扫描，在 299 nm 处有最大吸收，供试品溶液的紫外光谱与对照品溶液的紫外光谱应一致。

4. TLC 鉴定　取蟾酥粉末约 0.1 g 置于 25 ml 锥形瓶中，加二氯甲烷 10 ml 超声波提取 10 分钟后滤过，将滤液置于蒸发皿中蒸干，残渣用 1 ml 乙醇溶解，作为供试品溶液。分别取脂蟾毒配基对照品和华蟾酥毒基对照品各 2 mg 用 2 ml 乙醇溶解作为对照品溶液（全班共用）。将供试品溶液与对照品溶液分别点样于同一硅胶 G 板上，用环己烷－三氯甲烷－丙酮（4∶3∶3）为展开剂上行展开，取出，晾干，喷以 10% 硫酸乙醇溶液，加热至斑点显色清晰。供试品在与对照品相应的位置上应有相同的绿色斑点（脂蟾毒配基）和红色斑点（华蟾酥毒基）。

五、含量测定

1. 色谱条件　ODS C－18 反相色谱柱（150 mm×4.6 mm，5 μm），以 0.5% 磷酸二氢钾溶液－乙腈（50∶50）（用磷酸调节 pH 值为 3.2）为流动相；检测波长为 296 nm；柱温 40℃。

2. 供试品溶液制备　取于 80℃ 干燥 2 小时的蟾酥细粉约 25 mg，精密称定，置 50 ml 具塞锥形瓶中，精密加甲醇 20 ml，加热回流 1 小时，放冷，再称定重量，用甲醇补足减失的重量，摇匀，滤过，取续滤液，即得。

3. 对照品溶液制备（全班共用）　取华蟾酥毒基和脂蟾毒配基对照品各约 10 mg，精密称定，分别置于 100 ml 量瓶中，加甲醇稀释至刻度，摇匀，分别精密量取 5 ml 置于 10 ml 量瓶中，加甲醇稀释至刻度，摇匀，即得每 1 ml 含华蟾酥毒基、脂蟾毒配基 50 μg 的对照品溶液。

分别精密吸取上述两种对照品溶液与供试品溶液各 20 μl，注入液相色谱仪，测定。以外标一点法计算，本品含华蟾酥毒基（$C_{26}H_{34}O_6$）和脂蟾毒配基（$C_{24}H_{32}O_4$）的总量不得少于 6.0%。

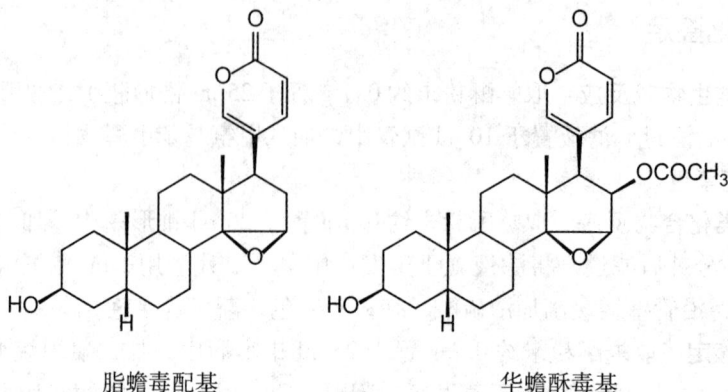

脂蟾毒配基　　　　　　　　　华蟾酥毒基

【报告要求】

1. 记录蟾酥药材的性状特征、显微化学鉴定结果。

2. 记述理化鉴别结果，绘制紫外光谱图和 TLC 色谱图。

3. 记述含量测定方法，提供 HPLC 色谱图及测定结果。

【思考题】

1. 生药蟾酥的基源是什么？有何主要功效？

2. 蟾酥主要含有哪些类型的化学成分？这些化合物主要有哪些药理作用？

Experiment 12　Identification of Animal Crude Drug —Toad Cake

Aim

1. Learn the morphologic characteristics of toad cake. Learn the physical and chemical i-dentification methods of toad cake. Learn the structure and operating method of HPLC. Learn the assay methods of toad cake.

Material

1. Animal specimens *Bufobufogargarizans* and *Bufomelanostictus Schneider*.

2. Crude drug andpowder of toad cake.

3. Standard reference material of bufogenin andcinobufagin.

Equipments and agents

1. Shimadzu 10Avp HPLC, UV detector, ODS C – 18 reverse phase column (150 mm × 4.6 mm, 5 μm), microinjector (25 μl), disposable filter (0.45 μm), sonicator, thin layer plate (5 cm × 20 cm), mortar, chromatographic tank, spoon, viltalight lamp, graduated cylin-der (10 ml, 20 ml, 100 ml), conical flasks with cover (50 ml), glass stick, two 25 ml coni-cal flasks, volumetric flask (25 ml, 100 ml), evaporating dish (with 10 cm of diameter), two beakers (100 ml), glass dropper, funnel, test tube (10 ml), capillary tube, absorbent cot-ton, filter paper, pin, glass slide and cover glassconical flasks.

2. Methanol, ethanol, acetonitrile (HPLC grade), redistilled water, monopotassium

phosphate, dilute glycerine, distilled water, concentrate sulfuric acid, dilute iodine solution, methanol, solid dimethylaminobenzaldehyde, chloroform, dichloromethane, acetic anhydride, ethanol, silica gel G, benzene, acetone, 1% CMC – Na solution and sea sand.

Methods

1. Original animals' identification

Observe the appearance characters of *Bufo bufo gargarizans* and *Bufo melanostictus Schneider*.

2. Morphologic identification

Observe the appearance of clumps and slices of toad cake.

Main points of observation: characteristics of shape, color, texture, fracture section and odor.

3. Microscopic identification

Take a bit of powder, test under microscope and identify as follows:

(1) Mount with dilute glycerine and irregular translucent fragments with sand – like solid can be seen.

(2) Mount with concentrated sulfuric acid, orange yellow or salmon pink appears, the fragments shrink gradually to form suborbicular transparent scraps with fissuaring texture surface and disappear gradually later.

(3) Mount with distilled water and add iodine solution, then observe, blue color should not appear (identifying starch).

4. Physical and chemical identification

1. Reaction of indole alkaloid　Take about 0.1 g of powder into 25 ml conical flask, add 5 ml of methanol and extract with supersonic for 5 min, filter, take the filtrate into 10 ml test tube, add a bit of dimethylaminobenzaldehyde and several drops of concentrated sulfuric acid and amethyst appears .

2. Reaction of steroid　Take about 0.1 g of powder into 25 ml conical flask, add 5 ml of dichloromethane and extract with supersonic for 5 min, evaporate the filtrate to dryness in evaporating dish, dissolve the residue with 1 ml of acetic anhydride, transfer into 10 ml tube, then add concentrated sulfuric acid along the wall, amethyst appears and turn to bluish – green gradually.

3. Vltraviolet spectra identtfication　Take about 0.1 g of powder into 25 ml conical flask, add 10 ml of dichloromethane and extract with supersonic for 10 min, evaporate 10 ml of the filtrate to dryness in evaporating dish, dissolve the residue with 5 ml of ethanol as a test solution. Dissolve 1 mg of bufogenin control article with 5 ml of ethanol as a control article solution. Measure the ultraviolet absorption spectrum of the test sample and control article solution, respectively, at the wave length 220 – 400 nm to get the maximum absorption at 299 nm; the test sample and the control article solution have the same ultraviolet spectra.

(4) TLC identification　Take about 0.1 g of powder into 25 ml conical flask, add 10 ml

of dichloromethane and extract with supersonic for 10 min, evaporate 10 ml of the filtrate to dryness in evaporating dish, dissolve the residue with 1 ml of ethanol as a test solution. Dissolve 2 mg of bufogenin and cinobufagin control article with 2 ml of ethonal as a control article solution, respectively (for the whole class). Apply the test sample and control article solution at the same silica gel G plate, develop with ascending method in developer of cyclohexane – acetone – acetone (4:3:3), take out, dry in the air, spray with 10% sulfuric acidethonal solution, heat to make the spot color is clear. The test solution should show the same green pot (bufogenin) or red pot (cinobufagin) with the same developing distance as that of the control article.

5. Assaying

(1) Chromatographic conditions   ODS C – 18 reverse phase column (150 mm × 4.6 mm, 5 μm), monopotassium phosphate – acetonitrle (50:50) as mobile phase, wave length 296 nm; column temperature 40℃.

(2) Preparation of test solution   weigh 25 mg of the powder dried for 2 h at 80℃ precisely into 50 ml conical flasks with cover, add 20 ml methonalprecisely, heating reflux for 1 h, cool, reweigh, then make up the weight loss reduction with methonal, shake and filter to get the subsequent filtrate.

(3) Preparation of standard solution (for the whole class)   weigh 10 mg of the standard reference of bufogenin andcinobufagin precisely into 100 ml volumetric flask, respectively, add methonalto the scale to shake, take 5 ml into a 10 ml measuring flask and add methanol to the scale to shake, to get the standard solutions at concentration 50 μg/ml of bufogenin andcinobufagin, respectively.

Take 20 μl of test solution and standard solution mentioned above precisely, injected into HPLC to analyse, respectively. The total contents of bufogenin ($C_{24}H_{32}O_4$) and cinobufagin ($C_{24}H_{32}O_4$) shouldnot be less than 6.0% according to external standard one point method.

Points in experiment report

1. Take notes of the morphologic characteristics and the results of microscopic chemical identification oftoad cake.

2. Record the results of physical and chemical identification of toad cake and draw its ultraviolet spectra and chromatogram of TLC.

3. Take notes of the method, chromatogram of HPLC and result of assaying.

Topics for thinking

1. What are the original animals of toad cake and its main effects?

2. What types of chemical composition are contained in toad cake? What are the main pharmacological effects of these compounds?

实验十三 矿物类生药——朱砂、石膏、信石的鉴定

【实验目的】

1. 掌握 朱砂、石膏、信石药材的性状、显微及理化鉴定方法。

2. 了解 朱砂、石膏、信石的含量测定方法。

【实验材料】

朱砂、石膏、信石药材及粉末。

【实验仪器与试剂】

1. 仪器 偏光显微镜、毛磁板、磁铁、铜片、试管、滴定管、小试管、铂丝、锥形瓶、滴定架、玻棒。

2. 试剂 盐酸、硝酸、氢氧化钠试液、碘化钾试液、氯化钡试液、醋酸铅试液、醋酸铵试液、硫酸、硝酸钾、1%高锰酸钾溶液、2%硫酸亚铁试液、硫酸铁铵指示液、0.1 mol/L硫氢酸铵溶液。

【实验内容】

一、性状鉴定

观察朱砂、石膏、信石生药材的性状。

观察要点：外形、颜色、气味、条痕、光泽、质地、硬度、解理、断口、透明度、有无磁性及相对密度。

二、显微鉴定

取朱砂、石膏、信石矿石，磨片后置偏光显微镜下观察。

观察要点：反射色、内反射色、偏光色、反射率、透光色、干涉色、消光性、晶轴、正光性、折射率、双折射率等。

三、理化鉴定

1. 朱砂

（1）取本品粉末用盐酸湿润后，在光洁的铜片上摩擦，铜片表面呈银白色光泽。加热烘烤，银白色消失。

（2）取本品粉末2 g，加盐酸－硝酸（3:1）的缓冲溶液2 ml溶解，蒸干，加水2 ml使溶解，滤过，制成供试液进行鉴定。

汞盐的鉴定：①取供试液0.2 ml，置小试管中，滴加氢氧化钠试液，产生黄色沉淀。②取供试液0.2 ml，置小试管中，滴加碘化钾试液，生成猩红色沉淀；继续滴加过量的碘化钾试液，沉淀溶解；加氢氧化钠试液碱化，加硫酸铵盐即生成红棕色沉淀。

硫酸盐鉴别：①取供试液0.2 ml，滴加氯化钡试液，生成白色沉淀；分离出沉淀，沉淀在盐酸或硝酸中均不溶解。②取供试液0.2 ml，滴加醋酸铅试液生成白色沉淀；分

离出沉淀，沉淀在醋酸铵试液或氢氧化钠试液中不溶解。

（3）取朱砂粉末少许，置带塞的试管中加热，变为黑色硫化汞；加碳酸钠共热，则变为金属汞球。

（4）取朱砂粉末少许，置开口试管中加热，产生二氧化硫气体及金属汞球。

2. 石膏

（1）取石膏一小块约 2 g，置具有小孔软木塞的试管中，灼烧，管壁有水生成，小块变成不透明体。

（2）取本品粉末 2 g，加稀盐酸 10 ml，加热溶解作为供试液。用铂丝蘸取供试液在无色火焰中燃烧，火焰呈砖红色。取供试液 1 ml，加甲基红指示液 2 滴，用氨试液中和，再滴加盐酸至恰呈酸性，加草酸试液生成白色沉淀；分离，沉淀不溶于醋酸，但可溶于盐酸。

（3）取本品粉末约 2 g，于 140℃烘 20 分钟，加水 1.5 ml，搅拌，放置 5 分钟，呈粘结状固体。

3. 信石

（1）本品于闭口管中加热，生成白色升华物（纯品 137℃升华）；

（2）水溶液为弱酸性，通硫化氢后产生三硫化二砷（As_2S_3）黄色沉淀。

四、含量测定

1. 朱砂 精密称定朱砂粉末约 0.3 g，置锥形瓶中，加硫酸 10 ml 与硝酸钾 1.5 g，加热使溶解，放冷，加水 50 ml 并加 1% 高锰酸钾溶液至显粉红色，再加 2% 硫酸亚铁溶液至红色消失后，加硫酸铁铵指示剂 2 ml，用硫氢酸铵液（0.1 mol/L）滴定，即得。每 1 ml 的硫氢酸铵液相当于 11.63 mg 的 HgS。本品含 HgS 不得少于 96.0%。

2. 石膏 精密称定石膏粉末约 0.3 g，置锥形瓶中，加稀盐酸 10 ml，加热使溶解，加水 10 ml，并加甲基红指示液 1 滴。滴加氢氧化钾试液至呈浅黄色，再继续多加 5 ml，加钙黄绿素指示液少量，用乙二铵四醋酸二钠液（0.05 mol/L）滴定至溶液的黄绿色荧光消失并显橙色，即得。每 1 ml 的乙二铵四醋酸二钠液相当于 8.608 mg 的 $CaSO_4 \cdot 2H_2O$。本品含 $CaSO_4 \cdot 2H_2O$ 不得少于 95.0%。

【报告要求】

1. 记录朱砂、石膏、信石药材的性状。

2. 记录朱砂、石膏、信石的显微鉴定结果。

3. 记录朱砂、石膏、信石的理化鉴别方法及结果。

4. 记录朱砂、石膏的含量测定方法及测定结果。

【思考题】

1. 朱砂、石膏、信石的基源及化学成分是什么？有何功效？

2. 朱砂、石膏、信石的理化鉴定各项的反应原理是什么？

3. 生石膏与熟石膏的化学成分、性状有何区别？药用功效有何不同？

4. 如何防治信石中毒？

Experiment 13　Identification of Mineral Crude Drugs— Cinnabar, Gypsum and Arsenolite

Aim

1. Learn the morphologic, microscopic, physical and chemical identification methods of cinnabar, gypsum and arsenolite.

2. Understand assaying methods of cinnabar, gypsum and arsenolite.

Material

Crude drugs and powders of Zhusha (cinnabar), Shigao (gypsum) and Xinshi (arsenolite)

Equipment and agents

1. Polarization microscope, white porcelain plate, magnet, copper slice, test tube, measuring glass, test tube, platinum filament, conical flask, titration hander and glass stick.

2. Hydrochloric acid, nitric acid, sodium hydroxide solution, kalium iodidum solution, barium chloride solution, lead acetate solution, ammonium acetate solution, sulfuric acid, kalium nitrate, 1% potassic permanganate, 2% ferrous sulfate solution, directive liquor of ammonium ferric sulfate and 0. 1 mol/L ammonium sulfydryl solution.

Methods

1. Morphologic identification

Observe the morphous of cinnabar, gypsum and arsenolite.

Main points of observation: shape, color, odor, streak, texture, hardness, cleavage, fracture, transparency, magnetism and specific gravity.

2. Microscopic identification

Take some of cinnabar, gypsum and arsenolite, grind them into powder and test under polarization microscope.

Main points of observation: reflected colour, internal reflected color, polarized light color, reflectivity, lucency color, interference color, extinction, crystallographic axis, positive photonasty, refractive index, birefraction, etc.

3. Physical and chemical identification.

(1) Cinnabar

① Take some of powder, moisten with hydrochloric acid, scrape on the glossy copper slice and then argentite color appears on the surface; the argentite color disappears in heating.

② Dissolve 2 g of powder with 2 ml of hydrochloric acid – nitric acid (3∶1) buffer solution and evaporate the solution to dryness, dissolve the residue with 2 ml of water and filter to make the sample solution for following tests.

Identification of mercury salts:

Ⅰ. Take 0. 2 ml of the test solution into a test tube and add sodium hydrate solution and yellow sediment is produced.

Ⅱ. Add potassium iodide into 0. 2 ml of the test solution and scarlet sediment is produced. Then, add excess potassium iodide to dissolve the sediment, alkalinize solution with sodium hydroxide, then add ammonium sulfate and reddish brown sediment appears.

Identification of sulphate:

Ⅰ. Take 0. 2 ml of the test solution, add barium chloride solution and white sediment appears; separate the sediment and add hydrochloric acid or nitric acid, but the sediment can't be dissolved.

Ⅱ. Take 0. 2 ml of the test solution, add lead acetate solution and white sediment appears; separate the sediment and add ammonium acetate or sodium hydroxide, but the sediment can't be dissolved.

③ Take a bit of powder, heat in test tube with stopper and the powder changes into black sulfide of mercury; heat in present of natrium carbonicum and the powder changes into mercury bead.

④ Take a bit of powder, heat in an opening tube and the gas of sulfur dioxide and mercury bead are produced.

（2）Gypsum

① Put 2 g of gypsum scraps into a test tube covered by cork with an eyelet, heat the test tube on fire and water vapour is seen on the tube wall and the scrap changes into opaque mass.

② Take 2 g of powder, add 10 ml of dilute hydrochloric acid, and dissolve in heating to be used as a sample solution. Dip a platinum filament in to the solution, burn on a colorless flame and a red flame is seen. Take 1 ml of the test solution, add 2 drops of methyl red indicator, neutralize with amonia solution, add hydrochloric acid until a proper acidity, add ethanedioic acid and white sediment appears; separate it and the sediment can't dissolve in the acetic acid, but in hydrochloric acid.

③Take 2 g of the powder, roast for about 20 min at 140℃ and add 1. 5 ml of water to shake, put aside for 5 min and stickiness solid appears.

（3）Arsenolite

① Heat in a close tube and white sublimate (pure substance sublimates at 137℃) appears.

② Its water solution is weak acidity so that yellow precipitate of arsenic trisulfide appears when be passed hydrogen sulfide.

4. Assaying

（1）Cinnabar Weigh about 0. 3 g of its powder precisely, put into a conical flask, add 10 ml of sulfuric acid and 1. 5 g of potassium nitrate, heat to make it dissolve, cool it, add 50 ml of water firstly, then 1% liquor potassic permanganate and pink red is shown; drop 2% ferrous sulfate solution until the red color disappears, add indicator of ammonium ferric sulfate and titrate with ammonio sulfydryl solution (0. 1 mol/L). Every 1 ml of ammonio sulfydryl solution corresponds to 11. 63 mg HgS. HgS contained in this mineral should not be less than 96. 0%.

（2）Gypsum Weigh about 0. 3 g of its powder precisely and put into the conical flask, add 10 ml of dilute hydrochloric acid, heat to make it dissolve, add 10 ml of water firstly, then 1 drop of indicator of methyl red solution and some potassium hydroxide solution to be light yellow, drop 5 ml more and then a bit of calcein indicator, titrate with disodium edetate (0.05 mol/L) until the yellow green fluorescence disappears. Every 1 ml of disodium edetate correspond to 8.608 mg $CaSO_4 \cdot 2H_2O$. The $CaSO_4 \cdot 2H_2O$ contained in the mineral should not be less than 95.0%.

Points in experiment report

1. Take notes of the morphous of cinnabar, gypsum and arsenolite.

2. Take notes of the results of microscopic identification of cinnabar, gypsum and arsenolite.

3. Take notes of the physical and chemical identification methods of cinnabar, gypsum and arsenolite.

4. Take notes of the results and methods of assaying of cinnabar and gypsum.

Topics for thinking

1. What are the originminerals and chemical compositions of cinnabar, gypsum, arsenolite, and their main effects?

2. What are the reaction principles of physical and chemical identification of cinnabar, gypsum and arsenolite?

3. What are the differences of chemical and appearance between gypsum and dried gypsum, and their effects?

4. How to prevent from poisoning of arsenolite?

实验十四　生药挥发油的提取及鉴定

【实验目的】

1. 通过苍术及白术根茎中挥发油的提取，掌握挥发油的特点、组成及性质。

2. 熟悉　挥发油的薄层层析鉴定方法及原理并比较苍术及白术挥发油成分的异同。

【实验材料】

茅苍术 [*Atractylodes lancea* (Thunb) DC.]，北苍术 [*A. chinensis* (DC.) Koidz.] 及白术 (*A. macrocephala* Koidz.) 的根茎。

【实验仪器与试剂】

1. 仪器　挥发油测定器一套、吸管、试管、层析槽、薄层板 (5 cm×20 cm)、毛细管、乳钵、荧光灯 (254 nm)、牛角勺。

2. 试剂　乙醚 (AR)、石油醚 (60～90℃，AR)、三氯甲烷 (AR)、无水硫酸钠、5%香草醛浓硫酸溶液、硅胶 G、0.5% CMC - Na 溶液。

【实验内容】

一、原理

在物质不溶于水的情况下，混合物的蒸气压等于组成该混合物的各物质的蒸气压总和。这样两种物质的混合物将在其蒸气压力之和等于外界压力的温度时开始沸腾。显然，每种物质可以在比其单独存在时的沸点低得多的温度即开始沸腾。

道尔顿分压定律：在一混合气体中，每种气体均能产生此混合气体的总压力的一部分，其压力大小与其在全部气体中所占的容积成正比。

$$P = P_1 + P_2 + P_3 + \cdots$$
$$P = P_1 \ (\ V_1 / \ V_{总}\ )$$

二、挥发油的提取

（1）称取北苍术、茅苍术或白术的粗粉 50 g，置挥发油测定器的底瓶中，加水 500 ml，振摇均匀后，接上接收管，连接冷凝器，从冷凝器的顶部加水至充满接收管并溢流入烧瓶为止。用直火加热至沸腾，保持微沸 2.0 小时，停止加热，放置片刻，待稍冷后取出接收管，冷却后备用。

（2）向接收管中加乙醚 2 ml，用吸管吸取醚层至另一干燥试管中，加入少许无水硫酸钠，留作点样用（图 2－35）。

三、挥发油的薄层鉴定

1. **检品** 茅术油、苍术油及白术油的乙醚液。

2. **支持剂** 硅胶 G～CMC。取硅胶 G 10 g，置乳钵中，加 0.5% 的 CMC～Na 溶液 30 ml，迅速研匀后铺板（此量可铺 5 cm×20 cm 板 5 块）。铺好后静置一夜，自然干燥后，于 105℃ 干燥半小时备用。

3. **展开剂** 乙酸乙酯～石油醚（15:85）。取展开剂约 15～20 ml，倒入层析槽中，盖好磨口盖。

4. **展开方式** 倾斜上行法。

5. **点样** 将检品溶液用毛细管仔细点加到已制备好的薄层板上，点的直径一般不大于 2～3 mm，点的间距一般为 1.5～2 cm，样品点加在距薄层板一端 1.5 cm 的起始线上，展开剂浸没薄层的起始线下边约为 0.5 cm。

6. **显色剂** 5% 香草醛浓硫酸溶液，喷雾（必要时烘烤）。

7. **结果** 观察与记录结果。

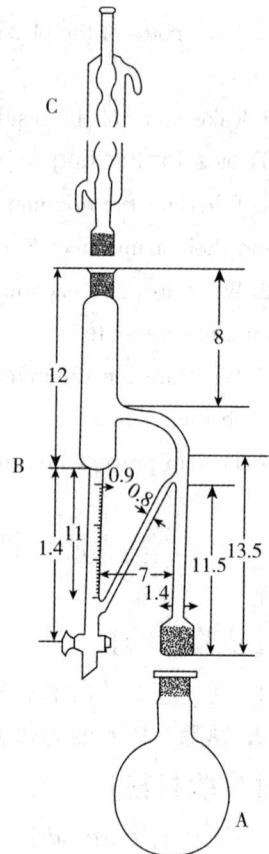

图 2－35 挥发油提取器

（单位：cm）

A. 圆底烧瓶

B. 挥发油测定器

C. 回流冷凝器

【报告要求】

1. 绘制实验装置图。

2. 记录薄层层析图谱并做讨论。

【思考题】

1. 什么是挥发油？挥发油在组成及性质上有什么特点？

2. 挥发油的提取方法有哪些？各有什么优缺点？

3. 薄层层析的原理是什么？影响因素有哪些？结合本次薄层层析实验讨论如何防止影响薄层层析结果的不利因素。

4. 白术与苍术的挥发油成分有什么不同？

Experiment 14　Extraction and Identification of Volatile Oil

Aim

1. Learn the characteristics, compositions and property of volatile oil through the extraction of atractylodes rhizome and largehead atractylodes rhizome.

2. Understard the identification method by TLC and the principle of volatile oil extraction, and compare the similarity and difference of the volatile oil composition of atractylodes rhizoma and largehead atractylodes rhizome.

Material

Maocangzhu (*Atractylodes lancea*), Beicangzhu (*A. chinensis*) and Baizhu (*A. macrocephala*).

Equipment and reagents

1. A set of volatile oil determination apparatus, measuring pipette, test tube, laminar analysis chute, thin layer plate (5 cm × 20 cm), capillary tube, mortar, fluorescent lamp (254 nm), spoon.

2. Diethyl ether (AR), petroleum ether (60 – 90℃, AR), chloroform (AR), natrii sulfas exsiccatus, 5% vanillin concentrated sulfuric acid solution, silica gel G, 0.5% CMC – Na solution.

Methods

1. Principle

When some substances can't dissolve in water, the vapor pressure of mixture composed by them is equal to the total vapor pressure produced by all the substances in the mixture. The mixture will start to boil at the temperature on which point the mixture's vapor pressure is equal to the surrounding's pressure. Obviously each substance in the mixture may boil at a much lower temperature than the point on which it boils separately.

Dalton law of partial pressure: in a mixture of gases, each gas can generate a portion of the total pressure and partial pressure magnitude is proportional to volume occupied by each portion.

$$P = P_1 + P_2 + P_3 + \cdots$$

$$P = P_1 \ (V_1 / V_{total})$$

2. Extraction procedure

(1) Put 50 g of coarse powder of atractylodes lancea or atractylodes rhizome or largehead atractylodes rhizome and 500 ml of water into flask of volatile oil determination apparatus, shake well, connect its receiving tube and condenser, and pour some water from the top of the condenser until the water is full of the receiving tube and overflows into the flask. Heat on great fire until boiling and keep ebullition for 2.0 hours, put aside until the receiving tube is cooled and unload.

(2) Pour 2 ml of diethyl ether to the receiving tube, imbibe the ether layer with a suctionpipe to another drying test tube, add a bit of natrii sulfas exsiccatus, and keep it for spotting.

3. Identification volatile oil by TLC

(1) Test article   The ether solution of oil extract of atractylodes lancea, atractylodes rhizome and largehead atractylodes rhizome.

(2) Support agent   Silica gel G - CMC. Put 10 g of silica gel G and 30 ml of 0.5% CMC - Na solution into mortar, grind well rapidly and plank (for five 5 cm × 20 cm plates). Put aside over night, air dried; dry for half an hour at 105℃ and reserved.

(3) Developing agent   Acetic ether - petroleum ether (15:85). Pour 15 - 20 ml into a chromatographic tank and cover it well.

(4) Developing way   Slope - ascending method.

(5) Spotting   Apply the test article solution on the prepared plate with a capillary tube, in general, the spot diameter should be less than 2 - 3 mm and the distance between two spots is 1.5 - 2 cm, and the starting line should be 1.5 cm apart from one end of the plate and the developer should immerse the plate 0.5 cm below the line.

(6) Chromogenic agent   0.5% vanillin concentrated sulfuric acid solution, spray (parch if necessary).

(7) Observe and record the results.

Points in experiment report

1. Draw the diagram of volatile oil determination apparatus.

2. Draw the thin layer chromatogram and discuss the results.

Topics for thinking

1. What is volatile oil and what are the characteristics of chemical constituents and property of volatile oil?

2. How many methods can be for the volatile oil extracting and what are the advantages and the disadvantages of each method?

3. What is the principle of TLC and what are its influence factors? Discuss how should we prevent from the disadvantages influenced TLC result according to this experiment?

4. What are the differences of the volatile oil composition between atractylodes rhizoma and largehead atractylodes rhizome?

实验十五　生药的理化鉴别

【实验目的】

1. 掌握　强心苷、皂苷、香豆精苷、生物碱、黄酮、多糖的定性反应及其原理；黄酮类的提取方法及薄层鉴别方法。

2. 通过对苦参的薄层鉴定，了解含生物碱类生药的薄层鉴定方法。

【实验材料】

1. 药材粉末　桔梗、洋地黄叶、白芷、苦参、黄芩粗粉、茯苓。

2. 标准品　苦参碱、氧化苦参碱、黄芩苷。

【实验仪器与试剂】

1. 仪器　电水浴、索氏提取器（50 ml）、磨口三角瓶（50 ml）、薄层板（5 cm × 20 cm 及 2.8 cm × 7.6 cm）、乳钵、牛角勺、试管（10 ml）、紫外灯、喷雾瓶、毛细管、滴管、层析缸、层析滤纸。

2. 试剂　三氯甲烷（AR 及工业用）、乙醇（工业用）、浓盐酸、1% 盐酸、碘化铋钾试液、碘化汞钾试液、碘 - 碘化钾试液、α - 萘酚试液、硫酸、甲醇（AR）、浓氨水、乙醚（AR）、Dragendorff 试剂、0.5 mol/L 草酸溶液、10% 醋酸铅溶液、镁粉、正丁醇、醋酸。

【实验内容】

一、强心苷的鉴别

Keller - Kiliani 反应　取洋地黄叶粉末约 0.5 g，加稀乙醇 30 ml，煮沸 2 分钟，放冷，加碱式醋酸铅试液 5 滴，滤过。滤液加三氯甲烷 10 ml，振摇，分取三氯甲烷层，蒸干。残渣加三氯化铁冰醋酸溶液（取冰醋酸 10 ml，加三氯化铁试液 1 滴制成）2 ml 溶解后，移置小试管中，沿管壁缓缓加入硫酸 2 ml，使成两液层，观察颜色变化，记录反应结果。（检查强心苷，α - 去氧糖的颜色反应）

二、皂苷的鉴别

取桔梗粉末约 0.5 g 置于 10 ml 试管中，加水 6 ml，煮沸，滤过，滤液加水至 6 ml，备用。

1. 泡沫反应　取滤液 2 ml，置于试管中，塞紧或以手指堵住管口，强烈振摇数分钟，观察是否可产生大量的泡沫，放置 10 分钟，记录泡沫的高度。

2. 溶血试验　取上述桔梗滤液 1 ml，加 1.8% NaCl 1 ml 及 2% 红细胞悬浮液 1 ml，振摇后放置数分钟，可见溶液渐变透明红色。

3. Liebermann 反应　取上述桔梗滤液 1 ml 于蒸发皿中，水浴蒸干，加醋酐 1 ml 使溶解，并转入小试管中，沿管壁滴加浓硫酸 1 ml，观察两液面交界处是否有紫色环出现。

三、香豆精苷的鉴别

异羟肟酸铁试验　取白芷 0.5 g，加甲醇 5 ml 热浸，滤过，浸出液加 7% 盐酸羟胺甲醇液与 10% 氢氧化钠溶液各数滴，在水浴上温热，冷后稀盐酸调 pH 至 3～4，加 1% 三氯化铁溶液，显红色至紫色。

四、生物碱的鉴别

（1）取苦参末（90 目）1 g，置 50 ml 磨口三角瓶中，加入 30 ml 三氯甲烷（内含浓氨水 0.3 ml）密塞，振摇后放置过夜，过滤得滤液备用。

（2）取上述滤液 10 ml，水浴上回收至干，残渣用 1% 盐酸 6 ml 溶解，过滤，取滤液分别置于 3 支试管中，分别加入碘化铋钾、碘化汞钾、碘-碘化铋钾，观察反应现象（生物碱沉淀反应）。

（3）取滤液 10 ml，浓缩后点于硅胶 G 板上，同时在对应的位置点苦参碱、氧化苦参碱标准品溶液作对照，用三氯甲烷-甲醇-浓氨水（5:0.6:0.2）展开。展开后立即喷雾显色，显色剂 Dragendorff 试剂，标记出斑点位置。

五、黄酮类的鉴别

（1）取黄芩粗粉（20 目）10 g 用滤纸筒装好。置索氏提取器中，以乙醚回流提取至提取液黄色（约 1 小时），收集提取液备用，残渣继续用 95% 乙醇回流提取 40 分钟，浓缩至适当体积（15 ml）备用。

（2）取黄芩乙醇提取液点于 0.5 mol/L 草酸溶液调制的硅胶 G 薄层上，以黄芩素标准品作对照，在三氯甲烷-甲醇（10:1）中展开，展距 15 cm，挥干展开剂后，以 2% 三氯化铝乙醇溶液喷雾，在紫外灯下观察，标记出斑点位置。

（3）将乙醇提取液点于层析滤纸上，用黄芩苷标准品作对照，以正丁醇-醋酸-水（6:2.5:1.5）作展开剂直立展开。挥干展开剂后，在紫外灯下观察并标记出斑点位置。

（4）HCl-Mg 反应。取黄芩生药乙醇提取液 6 ml，置于试管中，加入镁粉少许，然后滴加浓盐酸，显红色或紫红色（异黄酮、查尔酮、花色素类不显色）。

（5）金属盐类络合反应。取黄芩生药乙醇提取液 6 ml，置于试管中，加入 10% 醋酸铅 4～5 滴，生成有色络合物。

六、多糖类的鉴别

（1）取茯苓粗粉（20 目）10 g 置 100 ml 圆底烧瓶中，加入 5 倍量的水，回流提取 3 次，时间分别为 3、2、1 h。合并提取液，滤过，减压浓缩至 10 ml，搅拌下加入乙醇，使含醇量达到 80%，静置 12 h，离心，收集沉淀，加蒸馏水 50 ml 溶解煮沸，趁热过滤，滤液在搅拌下加入乙醇，使含醇量达到 80%，放置，析出褐色沉淀后，低温干燥，即得茯苓多糖粗品。

（2）Molish 试验。取上述茯苓多糖粗品 2 g，加入 α-萘酚数滴，摇匀，再沿管壁滴加浓硫酸，在液面交界处出现紫红色环。

【报告要求】

1. 记录各生药鉴定的操作及结果。

2. 绘薄层层析图谱，并写出结论。

3. 观察各类化合物的反应现象并记录。

【思考题】

1. 生药的理化鉴定方法有哪些？

2. 如何鉴定生药中含有的生物碱、黄酮苷、皂苷、强心苷、香豆精苷类及多糖类成分？

Experiment 15　Physical and Chemical Identification of Crude Drugs

Aim

1. Learn the qualitative reaction principle of flavonoid glycosides, saponins, cardiac glycosides and coumarin glycosides. Learn the extracting method and identification approaches by TLC of flavonoids.

2. Understand the identification method by TLC of alkaloids through the example of light-yellow sophora root.

Material

1. Drugs powders　coarse powder of Jiegeng (balloonflower toot), Yangdihuangye (foxglove leaf), Baizhi (dahuria angelica root), Kushen (lightyellow sophora root) and Huangqin (baical skullcap root) and *poria cocos*.

2. Standard articles　matrine, oxymatrine and baicalin.

Equipment and reagents

1. Hydroelectric bath, Soxhlet's apparatus (50 ml), frosting flask (50 ml), thin layer plates (5 cm × 20 cm and 2.8 cm × 7.6 cm), mortar, spoon, test tube (10 ml), ultraviolet lamp, spray bottle, capillary tube, dropping tube, chromatographic tank and filter paper for laminar analysis

2. Chloroform (AR or technica grade), ethanol (technica grade), concentrated hydrochloric acid, 1% hydrochloric acid, potassium heptaiodobismuthate solution, potassium mercuric iodide solution, I – KI solution, methanol (AR), ammonia water stronger, aether (AR), Dragendorff solution, 0.5 mol/L ethanedioic acid solution, 10% lead acetate solution, magnesium powder, *n* – butanol and acetic acid.

Methods

1. Identification of cardiac glycosides

Keller – Kiliani Reaction　Take 0.5 g of foxglove leaf fine powder, add 30 ml of diluted ethanol, boil for 2 min, cool it, add 5 drops of lead subacetate and filter. Add 10 ml of chloroform into the filtrate, shake, take the chloroform layer, and evaporate to dryness. Dissolve the residue with 2 ml of chloride ferric acetic acid solution (add 1 drop of chloride ferric into 10 ml of glacial acetic acid), move the solution into a test tube, drop 2 ml of sulphuric acid along the tube wall slowly to make the solution separated into two layers. Observe the color change and record the reaction results. (For identification of cardiac glycosides; the color reaction of α – deoxysaccharide).

2. Identification of saponins

Take about 0. 5 g of balloonflower root powder into a 10 ml test tube, add 6 ml of water, boil, filter, add water into the filtrate to 6 ml and reserve it.

(1) Foaming reaction   Take 2 ml of the filtrate into a test tube, block the opening and shake for some minutes. Observe the massive foam, put aside for 10 min and observe the foam height.

(2) Hemolysis test   Put 1 ml of the filtrate into a test tube, add 1 ml of 1. 8% NaCl and 1 ml of 2% erythrocyte suspension into the test tube, shake and put aside for some minutes to see the solution turn to transparent red gradually.

(3) Liebermann reaction   Take 1 ml of the filtrate into evaporating dish, evaporate to dryness in waterbath, resolve with 1 ml of acetic anhydride and transfer it into a test tube and drop into 1 ml of concentrated sulfuric acid. Observe whether the purple cycle appears between the two layers.

3. Identification of coumarin glycosides

Ferric hydroxamic acid reaction. Immerse 0. 5 g of dahuria angelica root into 5 ml of me thanol in heating, filter, add drops of 7% hydroxylamine hydrochloride methanol solution and 10% sodium hydrate solution into the leachate, warm in waterbath, modify pH value 3 – 4 when it is cooled and add 1% ferric chloride solution until red to purple appears.

4. Identification of lightyellow sophora root

(1) Put 1 g of lightyellow sophora root powder (90 mesh) and 30 ml of chloroform (containing 0. 3 ml of concentrated ammonia water) into a 50 ml flask, block it, shake and soak overnight, filter to get the soluble part and reserve it.

(2) Take 10 ml of the filtrate above, evaporate to dryness in waterbath, resolve the residue with 6 ml of 1% hydrochloric acid, filter, put the filtrate into three tubes and add potassium heptaiodobismuthate, potassium mercuric iodide and iodine – potassium heptaiodobismuthate, respectively and observe the reaction phenomenon (precipitation reaction of alkaloid).

(3) Take 10 ml of the filtrate and concentrate, apply it and the standard articles of matrine and oxymatrine as contrast on silica gel plate, develop the plate in chloroform – methanol – concentrated ammonia water (5: 0. 6: 0. 2). After developing, spray dragendorff reagent immediately and sign the the points position.

5. Identification ofbaical skullcap root

(1) Pack 10 g of baical skullcap root coarse powder (20 mesh) with a piece of filter pa-

per cylinder, put it into Soxhlet's apparatus, reflux with ether until the extract shows light yellow (for about 1 hour), take out the extract and reserve it; then reflux the residue with 95% ethanol for 40 min, concentrate the extract to proper volume (15 ml) and reserve it.

(2) Apply diethyl ether extract and the standard article baicalein on plate, on which silica gel mixed with 0.5 mol/L oxalic acid solution, develop in chloroform – methanol (10:1), and then spray 2% aluminum trichloride ethanol solution, observe under the uviol lamp and sign the points position.

(3) Apply the ethanol extract and the standard article baicalin on a piece of filter paper and develop in n – butanol – acetic acid – water (6:2.5:1.5), observe under uviol lamp and sign the points position.

(4) HCl – Mg reaction　Take 6 ml of ethanol extract into a tube, add some magnesium powder, then add some drops of hydrochloric acid until red to purple appears (No color appears for isoflavone, chalcone and anthocyanidin).

(5) Metal salts complexing reaction: take 6 ml of the ethanol extract into a tube, add some magnesium powder, then add 4 – 5 drops of 10% lead acetate solution to get colored complex.

6. Identification of polysaccharide

(1) Take 10 g of crude powder of *Poria coco*s (20 mesh) into a 100 ml round bottom flask, add five times of water, reflux for 3 times, 3 h, 2 h and 1 h for each time. Combine the extract, filter, vacuum concentration to 10 ml, add ethanol with stirring to left ethanol to 80%, stewing for 12 h, centrifuge and add 50 ml of distilled water to dissolve and boil, filter while hot, add ethanol into the filtrate with stirring to 80%, stewing, after brown sediment is separated out, cold drying and obtain polysaccharide of *Poria cocos*.

(2) Molish test: Take 2 g of polysaccharide of *Poria cocos* mentioned above, add some drops of alpha naphthol and shake, then add concentrated sulfuric acid along the tube's wall, the purplish red loop appears at the junction of two layers.

Points in experiment report

1. Record the identification operation and result of each crude drug.

2. Draw the thin – layer and paper chromatograms, and write out conclusions.

3. Observe and record the reaction phenomenon of various compounds.

Topics for thinking

1. What are the physical and chemical identification methods of crude drugs?

2. How to identify the crude drugs containing alkaloids, flavonoid glycosides, saponins, cardiac glycosides and coumarin glycosides?

实验十六   未知生药粉末的鉴定

【实验目的】

通过显微及理化方法对几种未知生药粉末进行鉴别。

【实验材料】

黄芩、大黄、川芎、苍术、黄柏、厚朴、肉桂、秦皮、黄连、苦参、人参、甘草、何首乌、半夏、川贝母、天麻、茯苓、猪苓、金银花、红花、洋金花、五味子、苦杏仁、薄荷、麻黄、大青叶、洋地黄叶、颠茄叶等生药粉末。

【实验仪器与试剂】

1. **仪器**   显微镜、载玻片、盖玻片、小玻棒、镊子、酒精灯、培养皿、纱布、滤纸、擦净纸、小试管、滴管、电水浴。

2. **试剂**   各种显微及化学鉴定试剂。

【实验内容】

随机抽取上述粉末中的几种，利用显微及理化方法加以鉴别。

【报告要求】

记录实验结果，绘出粉末显微特征图。

Experiment 16   Identification of Unknown Crude Drugs

Aim

Identify some unknown crude drugs powder by microscopic, physical and chemical methods.

Material

Drug powder：Huangqin（baical skullcap root）, Dahuang（rhubarb）, Chuanxiong（szechwan lovage rhizome）, Cangzhu（atractylodes rhizome）, Huangbai（amoorcorn tree bark）, Houpo（magnolia bark）, Rougui（Chinese cassia tree）, Qinpi（ash bark）, Huang lian（golden thread）, Kushen（lightyellow sophora root）, Renshen（ginseng）, GanCao（sweet root）, Heshouwu（fleeceflower root）, Banxia（pinelliae tuber）, Chuanbeimu（szechuan – fritillary bulb）, Tianma（tall gastrodia tuber）, Fuling（indian bread）, Zhuling（polyporus）, Jinyinhua（honeysuckle）, Honghua（safflower）, Yangjinhua（datura flower）, Wuweizi（Chinese magnoliavine fruit）, Kuxingren（bitter apricot seed）, Bohe（mint）, Mahuang（ephedra herb）, Daqingye（dyers woad leaf）, Yangdihuangye（foxglove leaf）and Dianqieye（belladonna leaf）.

Equipment and reagents

1. Microscope, slide, cover glass, glass stick, nippers, alcohol burner, culture capsule,

gauze, filter paper, lens paper, test tube, dropper and hydroelectric bath.

2. Various microscopic and chemical identification reagents.

Methods

Choose several powders above at random, identify by microscopic, physical and chemical methods.

Points in experiment report

Record experiment results, draw the diagrams of microscopic identification characteristics and write out the process of used physical and chemical reactions.

实验十七　开放性实验：药材标准的制定

【实验目的】

1. 掌握 几种药材的质量标准。

2. 了解 中药材药学研究的技术要求。

【实验材料】

黄芩、大黄、川芎、苍术、黄柏、厚朴、肉桂、秦皮、五加皮、黄连、苦参、人参、甘草、何首乌、半夏、川贝母、天麻、茯苓、猪苓、马勃、金银花、红花、洋金花、五味子、苦杏仁、薄荷、麻黄、大青叶、洋地黄叶、颠茄叶等生药饮片和粉末。

【实验仪器与试剂】

1. 仪器 显微镜、载玻片、盖玻片、小玻棒、镊子、酒精灯、培养皿、纱布、滤纸、擦净纸、小试管、滴管、电水浴、量瓶、量筒、薄层板、移液管，HPLC、UV、GC、MS 等仪器。

2. 试剂 各种显微及化学鉴定试剂。

【实验背景】

中药材的质量因外界因素的变化而受很大影响，为了保证临床用药或中成药新药研制中中药材质量的一致性和稳定性，《中国药典》2010 年版一部制定了中药材的质量标准，对其外观性状、组织特征、理化鉴别方法、杂质限量以及有关化学成分的含量测定都予以了规定。为了学习和掌握中药材质量标准的制定，设立此次实验。

中药材的质量标准项目有：名称、来源、性状、鉴别、检查、浸出物、含量测定、炮制、功能与主治、用法与用量、注意事项、贮藏等，具体说明如下。

1. **名称** 包括中文名称、汉语拼音、药材拉丁学名。

2. **来源** 包括原植（动）物的科名，原植（动）物的中文名、拉丁名、形态描述、生态环境、药用部位、采收季节和产地、加工等。

3. **性状** 主要指药材的形态、大小、色泽、表面色态、质地、断面、气味等。

4. **鉴别** 包括经验鉴别、显微鉴别、一般理化鉴别、色谱鉴别及其他鉴别。

5. **检查** 包括杂质、水分、总灰分、酸不溶性灰分、膨胀度、水不溶物、重金属、有害元素、农药残留量、SO_2残留、黄曲霉毒素等。

6. **浸出物** 对无法建立含量测定项的药材，可结合用药习惯、药材质地及化学成分等测定其浸出物的量。

7. **含量测定** 将药材中具有生理活性的主要化学成分，作为有效或指标性成分，建立含量测定项目，来评价药物的内在质量。

【实验内容】

任选所给实验材料中的一种药材，查阅文献资料，进行下列实验。

（1）鉴定所选药材的基原（并确定是否为药典品种）。

（2）描述所选药材的性状、进行显微特征的鉴别和描述。

（3）根据文献资料，进行该药材的理化鉴别实验和含量测定实验。

【报告要求】

根据实验及文献资料，起草制定所选药材的质量标准。

Experiment 17　Opening Experiment: Establish Quality Criteria of One Crude Drug

Aim

1. Master the quality criteria of some kinds of crude drugs.

2. Understand technique specifications of pharmaceutical research of Chinese crude drugs.

Material

Crude drug powder and cut crude drug: Huangqin (baical skullcap root), Dahuang (rhubarb), Chuanxiong (szechwan lovage rhizome), Cangzhu (atractylodes rhizome) Huangbai (amoorcorn tree bark), Houpo (magnolia bark), Rougui (Chinese cassia tree), Qinpi (ash bark), Wujiapi (slenderstyle acanthopenax bark), Huanglian (golden thread), Kushen (lightyellow sophora root), Renshen (ginseng), GanCao (sweet root), Heshouwu (fleeceflower root), Banxia (pinelliae tuber), Chuanbeimu (szechuan – fritillary bulb), Tianma (tall gastrodia tuber), Fuling (indian bread), Zhuling (polyporus), Mabo (puffball), Jinyinhua (honeysuckle), Honghua (safflower), Yangjinhua (datura flower), Wuweizi (Chinese magnoliavine fruit), Kuxingren (bitter apricot seed), Bohe (mint), Mahuang (ephedra herb), Daqingye (dyers woad leaf), Yangdihuangye (foxglove leaf) and Dianqieye (belladonna leaf).

Equipment and reagents

1. Microscope, slide, cover glass, glass stick, nippers, alcohol burner, culture capsule, gauze, filter paper, lens paper, test tube, dropper, water bath, measuring flask, measuring cylinder, thin layer plate, pipette, HPLC, UV, GC, MS equipments and etc.

2. Various of microscopic and chemical identification reagents.

Experiment background

The quality of Chinese materia medica can be greatly influenced by many external factors. In order to ensure its consistency and stability in the research of clinical medication and new Chinese patent medicine, Chinese Pharmacopoeia I made the quality criteria of some Chinese materia medica to prescribe their appearance property, tissue characters, physical and chemical identification methods, impurity limition and chemical composition assaying. To learn the establishing of medical material standard, we set up this experiment.

The items of medical material standard: denomination, origin, characteristic, identification, check, extract, assaying, processing, function and indication, application and dosage, announcements and storing, etc.. Details as follows.

(1) Denomination   Chinese name, Chinese spell and Latin name.

(2) Origin   family name of original plant (animal), Chinese name of original plant (animal), Latin name, appearance delineation, ecological environment, used part, collecting season, producing area and processing.

(3) Characteristic   morphous, size, color and luster, surface color, texture and odor, etc..

(4) Identification   experiential identification, microscopic identification, general physical and chemical identification and chromatographic identification, etc..

(5) Check   impurity, moisture, total ash, acid – insoluble ash, dilatability, water – insoluble substances, heavy metal, harmful element, pesticide residue, SO_2 residue and aflatoxin, etc..

(6) Extract   as to some kinds of medical materials, which can't be set up an assaying, we can determine their extract quantity according to their medication custom, texture and chemical compositions.

(7) Assaying   setting up assaying items by using the chief chemical composition with physiological activity as an indicatrix to evaluate internal quality of medical materials.

Methods

Choose one of the supplied drugs, refer to the literatures and carry out the following experiments.

(1) Identify its origin (and whether it corresponds to that in Chinese Pharmacopoeia).

(2) Describe its morphologic and microscopic characteristics.

(3) According to the literatures, carry out the experiments of physical and chemical identification and assaying.

Points in experiment report

Draft the quality criteria of your selected drug according to the experiment you did and literatures.

实验十八　生药川芎的 HPLC 指纹图谱分析

【实验目的】

1. 掌握　高效液相色谱仪的构造及使用方法。

2. 了解 生药的指纹图谱鉴定方法。

【实验材料】

1. 不同来源的川芎药材（8 批）。

2. 阿魏酸对照品。

【实验仪器与试剂】

1. 仪器 岛津 10Avp 型高效液相色谱仪，UV 检测器，ODS - C18 反相色谱柱（150 mm×4.6 mm，5 μm），微量进样器（25 μl），一次性滤器（0.45 μm），超声波仪，旋转薄膜蒸发仪，真空泵，50 ml 具塞锥形瓶，25 ml 茄形瓶，牛角匙，10 ml 量筒，漏斗，滤纸，滴管，分析天平，25 ml 量瓶，10 ml 量瓶，100 ml 分液漏斗

2. 试剂 甲醇（色谱纯），重蒸水，冰醋酸（分析纯）。

【实验原理】

中药指纹图谱系指中药经适当处理后，采用一定的分析手段和仪器检测，得到的能够标示该中药特性的共有峰的图谱。目前中药指纹图谱的研究方法主要有色谱指纹图谱、光谱指纹图谱以及生物指纹图谱等，较为常用的为 HPLC 指纹图谱。通过 HPLC 指纹图谱中主要特征峰的相对保留时间及含量或比例的制定和比对，来有效地控制中药材的真伪优劣以及中药产品质量，保证中药质量的相对稳定。

【实验内容】

4 人/组，共分 8 组，每组各测试 1 批样品。

一、样品溶液的制备

称取川芎药材粉末 2.0 g（过 40 目筛），分别置于 50 ml 具塞锥形瓶中，加入 40 ml 甲醇，于超声波振荡器中超声提取 30 分钟，滤过。滤液减压浓缩至干，残留物以 20 ml 蒸馏水溶解，混悬液用乙酸乙酯（20 ml，20 ml，10 ml）萃取 3 次，合并萃取液，减压浓缩至干。残渣加适量甲醇溶解，转移至 10 ml 量瓶中，所用容器用甲醇润洗 3 遍，合并润洗液至上述 10 ml 量瓶中，加甲醇至刻度，摇匀，即得。取适量样品溶液，用 0.45 μm 滤器滤过，取续滤液进行分析。

二、标准品溶液的制备

精密称取阿魏酸对照品 10.0 mg，置于 100 ml 棕色量瓶中，加甲醇溶解，定容，配制成浓度为 0.10 mg/ml 的对照品储备液。分别精密移取 0.1、2、4、6、8 和 10 ml 对照品储备液置于 10 ml 棕色量瓶中，分别用甲醇稀释至刻度，摇匀，即得浓度分别为 1、20、40、60、80 和 100 μg/ml 的对照品工作液。

三、色谱条件

流动相：甲醇 - 水 - 冰醋酸（30∶70∶0.5，*V/V/V*）

检测波长：276 nm。

流速：1.0 ml/min。

室温测定：____℃。

进样量：10 μl。

四、HPLC 指纹图谱的建立

（1）用流动相平衡高效液相色谱仪，直至基线平稳。取微量进样器吸取川芎样品溶液 10 μl，进样，按上述色谱条件进行色谱分析，色谱图记录时间 60 分钟，得到川芎有效部位的 HPLC 图谱。

（2）取微量进样器吸取 20 μg/ml 阿魏酸对照品溶液 10 μl，进样，按上述色谱条件进行色谱分析，色谱图记录时间 60 min，得到对照品 HPLC 图谱。

（3）共有峰的确定。收集 8 组的测试数据。以阿魏酸峰的保留时间为基准，计算其余各峰的相对保留时间（$\alpha = t_i / t_阿$）（注：t_i 为各主要色谱峰的保留时间，$t_阿$ 为阿魏酸峰的保留时间）。相对保留时间（α）的相对偏差小于 3%，可以确定为共有峰。

（4）收集 8 组的测试数据。以阿魏酸峰的峰面积为基准，计算其余各共有峰的相对峰面积值（$A_R = A_i / A_阿 \times 100\%$）及相对偏差（注：$A_i$ 为各共有色谱峰的峰面积，$A_阿$ 为阿魏酸峰的峰面积）。确定各共有峰的相对比例。

（5）通过中药指纹图谱计算机辅助相似度评价软件，对 8 组的图谱及数据进行综合评价，得到川芎药材有效部位的标准指纹图谱。

五、生药川芎的含量测定

1. 标准曲线的建立 精密吸取阿魏酸对照品工作液各 10 μl，以上述色谱条件进行色谱分析，以阿魏酸溶液浓度为横坐标（X），相应峰面积为纵坐标（Y），绘制标准曲线。

2. 计算含量 用外标法计算所制备川芎样品中阿魏酸的含量。

【报告要求】

1. 记录本组测试得到的川芎 HPLC 指纹图谱。

2. 标记川芎 HPLC 指纹图谱中共有峰的相对保留时间。

3. 计算共有峰的相对峰面积，给出共有峰的相对比例。

4. 记录生药川芎的含量测定结果。

5. 讨论。

【思考题】

1. 简述 HPLC 仪的结构及各部分功能。

2. 用于中药指纹图谱研究的药材（药品）来源有什么要求？

3. 中药指纹图谱有什么优缺点？

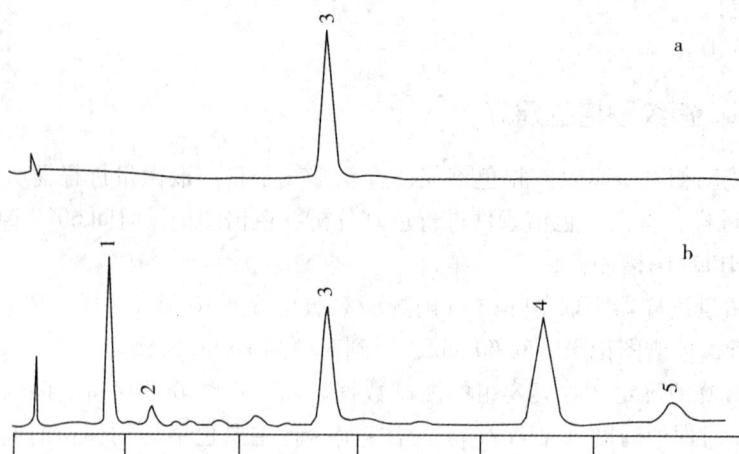

图 2 - 36　川芎药材有效部位的标准指纹图谱
a. 对照品溶液　b. 供试品溶液
1 ~ 5. 供试品溶液中各成分的色谱峰　3. 阿魏酸

Experiment 18　HPLC Finger Print Analysis of Szechwan Lovage Rhizome

Aim

1. Learn the constitution and using method of high performance liquid chromatograph.

2. Understand the identification method by using HPLC finger print of crude drugs.

Material

1. The crude drugs of Szechwan lovage rhizome from eight different habitats.

2. Reference substance of ferulaic acid.

Equipment and reagents

1. High performance liquid chromatograph: Shimadzu 10Avp, UV detector, ODS – C 18 reversed phase chromatography column (150 mm × 4. 6 mm, 5 μm), microsyringe (25 μl), one – off filter (0. 45 μm), ultrasonoscope, rotation film evaporator, vacuum pump, 50 ml conical flask with block, 25 ml eggplant shaped flask, horn spoon, 10 ml graduated cylinder, funnel, filter paper, dropper, analytic balance, 10 ml measuring flask, 25 ml measuring flask and 100 ml separating funnel.

2. Methanol (chromatographic pure), redistilled water, ethyl acetate and glacial acetic acid (analytical pure).

Principles of experiment

Finger print of Chinese crude drug refers to the common peaks atlas expressed its characteristics, which is obtained by some kinds of analysis methods and detecting equipments after the drug is processed by proper ways. At present, the main researching methods of fingerprint include chromatographic, spectrum and biology atlases, etc. HPLC finger print is a commonly used one. With the establishment and comparison of relative retention time, content and proportion of the main characteristic peaks, we can effectively control the authenticity and products quality of Chinese crude drug.

Methods

8 groups, 4 people in each group responsible for measuring of a batch of the drugs.

1. The preparation of sample solution

Put 2.0 g of the crude drug powder (40 screen mesh) and 40 ml of methanol into a conical flask, extract for 30 min in an ultrasonic oscillator, filter and concentrate the filtrate to dryness under reduced pressure, dissolve the residue with 20 ml of distilled water, then extract the suspension with acetic ether for three times (20, 20, 10 ml), combine the extract and condense to dryness under reduced pressure, dissolve the residue with appropriate amount of methanol, transfer into a 10 ml measuring flask, rinse all the containers used with methonal for 3 times, combine rinse solution into the 10 ml measuring flask above, and add methanol to the scale to shake. Take appropriate amount of test sample, filter with 0.45 μm filter, and the subsequent filtrate was used to analyse.

2. Preparation of standard solutions

Weigh 10.0 mg of the standard preparation of ferulaic acid precisely, put it into a 100 ml brown measuring flask, dissolve with methanol and metered volume to get the standard stock solution at the concentration of 0.10 mg/ml. Transfer 0, 1, 2, 4, 6, 8 and 10 ml standard stock solution into 10 ml brown measuring flask, respectively, add methanol and metered volume to get the standard working solutions at the concentration of 1, 20, 40, 60, 80 and 100 μg/ml.

3. Chromatographic condition

Mobile phase: methanol – water – glacial acetic acid (30:70:0.5, *V/V/V*).

Wave length for detection: 276 nm.

Flow rate: 1.0 ml/min.

Determining at room temperature: ＿＿℃.

Sample size: 10 μl.

4. Establishment of HPLC finger print

(1) Counterpoise the high performance liquid chromatograph by flowing mobile phase until the baseline is stable. Imbibe 10 μl of the sample solution with microsyringe and inject; measure according to the above – mentioned chromatographic condition to get the HPLC chromatogram of active part of Szechwan lovage rhizome.

(2) Imbibe 10 μl of ferulaic acid standard solution at concentration of 20 μg/ml with microsyringe, measure according to the above – mentioned chromatographic condition with running time of the chromatogram 60 min, and get the HPLC chromatogram of the standard article.

（3）Definition of the common peaks： collect the test data of the total eight groups. Choose the retention time of the ferulaic acid peak asa reference，calculate the relative retention time of the other peaks $\alpha = t_i/t_F$ （comments： t_i the retention time of the main chromatographic peaks，t_F the retention time of the ferulaic acid peak）. If the RSD of relative retention time （α）is less than 3%，we can regard it as the common peak.

（4）Collect the test data of the total eight groups. Choose the peak area of ferulaic acid as a reference，calculate the relative peak area of other common peaks （$A_R = A_i/A_F \times 100\%$）and their RSD （comments： A_i is the peak area of each common peak，A_F isthe peak area of ferulaic acid）. Determine the relative ratio of each common peak.

（5）Standard finger print atlas of the active part of Szechwanlovage rhizome is obtained by appraising all the atlases and data synthetically by the computer – assisted similarity evaluation software of Chinese materiamedica finger print.

5. Determination of Szechwan lovage rhizome

（1）Establishment of Standard Curve. Imbibe 10 μl of standard working solutions separately with microsyringe，measure according to the above – mentioned chromatographic condition. The concentration of ferulaic acid is taken as abscissa （X），and the corresponding peak area is taken as ordinate （Y）to calculate the standard curve.

（2）Calculating the content of ferulaic acid in Szechwan lovage rhizome samples by external standard method.

Points in experiment report

1. Record the HPLC finger print atlas of Szechwanlovage rhizome.

2. Record therelative retention time of all common peaks in the HPLC finger print atlas.

3. Calculate the relative peak and proportion area of common peaks.

4. Record the results of content determination.

5. Discussing.

Topics for thinking

1. What are the constitution and function of each part inhigh performance liquid chromatograph?

2. What's the requirement for the origin of crude drugs used for HPLC finger print research?

3. What are advantages and disadvantages of HPLC finger print of Chinese materia medica?

实验十九　PCR – RFLP 法鉴定生药川贝母

【实验目的】

1. 熟悉　植物 DNA 的提取方法；熟悉 PCR 的基本操作及原理。

2. 了解　DNA 分子标记法在生药鉴定中的应用。

【实验材料】

1. 川贝母对照药材，松贝、青贝、炉贝、浙贝母、平贝母、新疆贝母、丽江山慈菇。

2. PCR引物（上游引物，30 μmol/L）：5′ CGTAACAAGGTTTCCGTAGGTGAA 3′和5′ GCTACGTTCTTCATCGAT 3′。

【实验仪器与试剂】

1. 仪器 全自动基因扩增仪，高速离心机，多功能紫外透射仪，微量移液器（1~20 μl、20~200 μl、100-1000 μl），吸头（10 μl、200 μl、1000 μl），1.5 ml Eppendorf离心管，200 μl PCR管，电泳仪，镊子，乳钵，研棒，水浴锅，250ml三角瓶，分析天平，恒温培养箱，吸水纸，制冰机。

2. 试剂 新型广谱植物基因组DNA快速提取试剂盒，RNase（10 mg/ml），TE缓冲液（pH 7.6的100 mmol/L Tris-HCl，pH 8.0的10 mmol/L EDTA），1×TAE缓冲液（0.04 mol/L Tris-乙酸，0.001 mol/L EDTA），高保真Taq酶（5 U/μl），10×扩增缓冲液，二氯化镁（25 mmol/L），琼脂糖，dNTPs（10 mmol/L），10×酶切缓冲液，Gel-Red，上样缓冲液，75%乙醇，灭菌超纯水，蒸馏水，*Sma* I（10 U/μl），DNA Marker（0.5 μg/μl）。

【实验原理】

1. **多聚酶链式反应**（polymerase chain reaction，PCR） 是一种快速体外DNA片段扩增技术。它以待扩增的两条DNA链为模板，由一对人工合成的寡核苷酸作为介导，通过DNA聚合酶促反应，在体外进行特异DNA序列扩增。其过程包括模板变性（denature）、引物退火（annealing）和用DNA聚合酶延伸（elongation）退火引物在内的重复循环阶段，使末端被引物5′端限定的特异性片段成指数形式积累。

引物在PCR过程中具有至关重要的作用，通过选择物种特异性引物，可以特异扩增单一物种的特定基因片段，从而达到快速、准确鉴别的目的。

2. **限制性内切酶片段长度多态性**（Restriction Fragment Length Polymorphism，RFLP） 是利用限制性内切酶能识别DNA分子的特异序列并切开的特性，将不同物种DNA切割成大小不等、数量不同的片段，这些DNA限制性酶切片段经电泳分离、Southern印迹法可显示出RFLP谱带。不同物种的DNA由于酶切位点数量和长度不同，而使电泳谱带表现出不同程度的多态性。

【实验内容】

一、DNA模板的快速提取

（1）取川贝母对照药材0.1 g，依次用75%乙醇1 ml、灭菌超纯水1 ml清洗，吸干表面水分，置乳钵中研磨成极细粉。

（2）取20 mg，置1.5 ml离心管中，用植物基因组DNA快速提取试剂盒提取DNA。加入缓冲液AP1 400 μl和RNase溶液（10 mg/ml）4 μl，涡漩振荡，65°C水浴加热10分钟，加入缓冲液AP2 130 μl，充分混匀，冰浴冷却5分钟，高速离心（14000 rpm）

10 分钟；吸取上清液转移入另一离心管中，加入 1.5 倍体积的缓冲液 AP3/E，混匀，加到吸附柱上，离心（13000 r/min）1 分钟，弃去过滤液，加入漂洗液 700 μl，离心（12000 r/min）30 秒，弃去过滤液；再加入漂洗液 500 μl，离心（12000 r/min）30 秒，弃去过滤液；再离心（13000 r/min）2 分钟，取出吸附柱，放入另一离心管中，加入 50 μl 洗脱缓冲液，室温放置 3~5 分钟，离心（12000 r/min）1 分钟，将洗脱液再加入吸附柱中，室温放置 2 分钟，离心（12000 r/min）1 分钟；取洗脱液，作为供试品溶液，置 4℃ 冰箱中备用。

（3）取川贝母商品药材及其他伪品药材，按上述步骤分别提取 DNA。

二、PCR 扩增反应

在无菌的 200 μl PCR 管内加入以下反应物。

反应物	体积/ml
无菌超纯水	21.8
10×扩增缓冲液	3
dNTP	0.6
引物	各 0.5
模板 DNA	1
二氯化镁	2.4
高保真 Taq 聚合酶	0.2

混匀，简短离心。将 PCR 管置于全自动基因扩增仪中，按以下程序进行扩增：95℃ 预变性 4 min；循环反应 30 次：95℃ 30 s，55℃ 30 s，72℃ 30 s；72℃ 延伸 5 min。

另取无菌超纯水为模板，同法上述 PCR 反应操作，作为空白对照。

三、RFLP 反应

取 PCR 反应液，置 200 μl PCR 管中，进行酶切反应，反应总体积为 20 μl，反应体系包括 10×酶切缓冲液 2 μl，PCR 反应液 6 μl，*Sma* Ⅰ 0.5 μl，无菌超纯水 11.5 μl，酶切反应在 30℃ 反应 2 小时。

四、电泳检测

1. 琼脂糖凝胶的制备

（1）在已加有 100 ml 1×TAE 电泳缓冲液的三角瓶中加入准确称量的琼脂糖粉 1.5 g，使其浓度为 1.5%（W/V）。在沸水浴中加热至琼脂糖溶解。

（2）使溶液冷却至约 60℃。加入 GelRed 至终浓度为 0.5 μg/ml，充分混匀。

（3）将剩余的温热琼脂糖溶液倒入胶膜中。凝胶厚度在 3~5 mm 之间。在胶膜上放置梳子。

（4）在凝胶完全凝固后（于室温放置 30~45 min），小心移去梳子，将凝胶放入电泳槽中。

（5）在电泳槽中加入恰好没过胶面约 1 mm 深的足量 1×TAE 电泳缓冲液。

2. 电泳 DNA Marker 上样量 2 μl，并取对照药材、商品药材、伪品药材及空白对照酶切反应液各 8 μl，与 5 μl 上样缓冲液混匀后，慢慢加至样品槽中。盖上电泳槽并通电（采用 2.5 V/cm 的电压），开始电泳。

电泳结束后，切断电流，从电泳槽上拔下电线，打开槽盖。在紫外透射仪上检测并拍照。记录实验结果。

【报告要求】

1. 记录川贝母药材及其伪品的 PCR – RFLP 反应物琼脂糖凝胶图谱。
2. 实验结果、结论及讨论。

【思考题】

1. PCR – RFLP 的基本原理？
2. DNA 分子标记在生药鉴定中的作用？

Experimert 19　Identification of Szechwan – fritillary bulb with PCR – RFLP

Aim

1. Familiar with the extraction methods of plant DNA. Familiar with the basic operation and principle of PCR.

2. Understand the application of DNA molecular marker in identification of crude drugs.

Material

1. Standard crud drug of Szechwan – fritillary bulb, Szechwan – fritillary bulbs, Fritillaria Thunbergii Bulbus, Fritillaria Ussuriensis Bulbus, bulbs of *Fritillaria walujewii*, bulbs of *Iphigenia indica*.

2. PCR primer (Forward primer, 30 mmol/L): 5′ CGTAACAAGGTTTCCGTAGGTGAA 3′ and reverse primer 5′ GCTACGTTCTTCATCGAT 3′.

Equipment and reagents

1. PCR, high – speed centrifuge, multifunctional ultraviolet transilluminator, micropipette (1 – 20 μl, 20 – 200 μl, and 100 – 1000 μl), 1.5 ml Eppendorf tube, 200 μl PCR tube, electrophoresis apparatus, nippers, pestle, grinding rod, water bath, 250ml triangular bottle, analytical balance, incubator, absorbent paper, ice maker.

2. Rapid Extraction Kit of Plant Genome DNA, RNase (10 mg/ml), TE buffer (pH 7.6 100 mmol/L Tris – HCl, and pH 8.0 10 mmol/L EDTA), 10 × Amplification buffer (500 mmol/L KCl, 100 mmol/L Tris – HCl, pH 8.3, at room temperature, 15 mmol/L $MgCl_2$, 0.1% gelatin), 1 × TAE buffer (0.04 mol/L Tris – HAc, 0.001 mol/L EDTA), High fidelity Taq enzyme (5 U/μl), agarose, dNTPs (10 mmol/L), GelRed (10 mg/ml), $MgCl_2$ (25 mmol/l), 10 × Enzyme digestion buffer, loading buffer, *Sma* I (10　U/μl), DNA Marker (0.5 μg/μl), 75% ethanol and distilled water.

Principles of experiment

1. PCR

PCR (polymerase chain reaction) is the technology thatamplifies specific DNA sequence quickly *in vitro* by the enzymatic reaction of DNA polymerase. Target DNA is as template and a pair of synthetic oligonucleotides are as primers. The procedure includes the recycling of template denature, primer annealing and elongation of annealed primer by DNA polymerase to make the specific fragments whose terminal is limited by 5' – terminal of primer accumulate in index number. Primers play an important role in the process of PCR. By selecting species – specific primers, gene fragments of a single species can be specifically amplified to achieve rapid and accurate identification.

2. RFLP

RFLP (Restriction Fragment Length Polymorphism) is a technique that exploits variations in homologous DNA sequences. It refers to a difference between samples of homologous DNA molecules from differing locations of restriction enzyme sites, and to a related laboratory technique by which these segments can be illustrated. In RFLP analysis, the DNA sample is broken into pieces (digested) by restriction enzymes and the resulting restriction fragments are separated according to their lengths by gel electrophoresis.

Methods

1. Extraction of DNA template

(1) Use 1 ml of 75% ethanol and then 1 ml of sterile ultra pure water to wash 0.1 g of standard crud drug of Szechwan – fritillary bulb, and then dry the surface water and grind it into very fine powder.

(2) Take 20 mg powder into 1.5 ml centrifugal tube, and extract DNA with plant genome DNA rapid extraction kit. Add buffer AP1 400 μl and RNase solution (10 mg/ml) 4 μl, then 65 °C water bath heating for 10 min. Add buffer AP2 130 μl, mixed well, then cooling for 5 minutes in ice bath. After centrifuged (14000 rpm) for 10 min; transfer supernatant to another centrifugal tube, add 1.5 times volume buffer AP3/E, mixed well, then add to adsorption column, centrifuge (13000 rpm) for 1 min. Discard the filtrate, add 700 μl rinse solution, centrifuge (12000 rpm) for 30 seconds, discard the filtrate; add 500 μl rinse solution, centrifuge (12000 rpm) for 30 seconds, and discard the filtrate. Then centrifuge (13000 rpm) for 2 min, take out the column and put it in a new centrifugal tube. Add 50 μl elution buffer, place it at room temperature for 3 to 5 minutes, centrifuge (12000 rpm) for 1 min, add the eluent to the column, place it at room temperature for 2 minutes, and centrifuge (12000 rpm) again for 1 minute; take the eluent as the sample solution and keep it in 4 °C.

(3) The DNA of commercial or counterfeit Szechwan – fritillary bulb was extracted according to the above steps.

2. PCR amplification reaction

Add the following reagents into sterile200 μl PCR tube.

Reactant	Volume / Ml
Sterile water	21. 8
10 × amplification buffer	3
dNTP	0. 6
Primer	0. 5 (each primer)
DNA template	1
MgCl$_2$	2. 4
High fidelity Taq enzyme	0. 2

Mix well and then put the PCR tube into the automatic gene amplification instrument and amplify as the following procedure: react at 95°C for 4 min, then carry out 30 cycles, in each includes 30 s denaturalization at 95°C, 30 s annealing at 55°C, 30 s polymerization at 72°C and elongate at 72°C for 5 min.

3. RFLP reacion

ThePCR product is placed in a 200 μl PCR tube for enzymatic digestion. The total volume of the enzyme digestion reaction is 20 μl consisting 10 × digestion buffer 2 μl, PCR product 6 μl, *Sma* Ⅰ 0. 5 μl, sterile ultra – pure water 11. 5 μl, and digestion reaction is carried out at 30 °C for 2 hours.

4. Agarose gel electrophoresis

（1）Preparation of agarose gel

① Seal rims of the clean and dry glass plate with autoclaving indicating paper tapes to form a gel membrane. Put the gel membrane on the worktable plane.

② Add accurately weighed agarose powder into triangular flask with proper electrophoresis buffer to make its concentration as 1. 5% (W/V) . Heat in boiling waterbath until the agarose is dissolved.

③ Cool the solution to 60℃ and add Gelred to make the final concentration at 0. 5 μg/ml and mix thoroughly.

④ Imbibe a little agarose solution to seal gel membrane rim, wait until it is congealed. Lay a comb at 0. 5 – 1. 0mm from the bottom.

⑤ Pour the remaining lukewarm agarose into the gel membrane to make its thickness as 3 – 5mm.

⑥ When the gel is completely congealed (at room temperature for 30 – 45 min) , dislodge the comb and autoclaving paper tape carefully, and put the gel into an electrophoresis chamber.

⑦ Add sufficient 1 × TAE electrophoresis buffer over the gel surface 1mm rightly.

（2）Electrophoresis　Take 2 μl of DNA Marker and 8 μl of digested products of standard crud drug, commercial crud drug, counterfeit crud drug, and control sample separately, put into the sample gutter slowly, cover it and switch on (voltage 2. 5 V/cm) , and the electrophoresis begins.

When electrophoresis is completed, switch off, unfold the cover, determine andtake photographs under ultraviolet lamp.

Points of experiment report

1. Provide the PCR – RFLP gel electrophoresis map.

2. Record the experiment results and discussions.

Topics for thinking

1. What is the basic principle of PCR – RFLP?

2. What is the role of DNA Molecular Markers in crud drug identification?

实验二十　药用植物园及标本室实习

【实验目的】

1. 通过对生长期的植物形态观察，尤其是花形态的观察，进一步体会植物的分类。

2. 了解不同科的有代表性的植物 30 种，记住主要特征，进一步体会科的概念，并掌握 10 个科的特征。

3. 通过生药标本室实习，进一步掌握重点药的性状鉴定特征及方法。

【实验内容】

一、药用植物园实习

分成 2 组，由任课老师指导熟悉下列植物的特征，并做好观察记录，写出对植物分类的体会。重点观察主要科（＊）的植物特征。

（一）蕨类植物　Pteridophyta

蕨类植物是高等植物中具有维管组织，但比较低级的一类群。具有明显的世代交替，孢子体和配子体都能独立生活，孢子体发达。陆生、附生或水生。常见的蕨类植物体（孢子体）有根、茎、叶的分化。根为不定根，茎多为根状茎，常被毛茸或鳞片。叶多由根茎生出，根据叶的起源和形态特征，分为大型叶和小型叶。孢子囊单生或聚成孢子囊群，分布于枝的顶端球状或穗状的孢子叶的背面、边缘或集生，多数孢子囊聚集成形状多样的孢子囊穗，有或无囊群盖。孢子大多数为同型；少数为异型，分别生于大小孢子囊中。

现有蕨类植物约 12000 种，以热带、亚热带分布最多，多为草本植物。我国约有 2600 种，可供药用的有 455 余种。

（1）卷柏科 Stlaginellaceae

卷柏 *Selaginella tamariscina*（Beauv）Spr.

（2）木贼科 Equisetaceae

问荆 *Equisetum arvense* L.

木贼 *E. hyemale*（L.）Boern.

（3）鳞毛蕨科 Dryopteridaceae

贯众 *Cyrtomium fortonei* J. Sm.

粗茎鳞毛蕨 *Dryopteris crassirhizoma* Nakai.

（4）水龙骨科 Polypodiaceae

石韦 *Pyrrosia petiolosa*（Christ）Ching

（二）裸子植物　**Gymnospermae**

孢子体（植物体）发达，多为常绿木本植物，主根发达，茎有形成层和木栓形成层可次生生长，维管素排列成环状，木质部大多为管胞，韧皮部中有筛胞而无半胞。配子体微小，非常退化，完全寄生于孢子体上。雄配子体内的精子与雌配子体内的卵细胞结合时不需以水为媒介。花常缺少花被，胚珠裸露。

古代，裸子植物与蕨类植物是非常繁茂的植物群，后来衰退，多数被绝灭，现有12 科 71 属近 800 种，我国有 11 科 41 属 236 种，药用有 10 科 25 属 100 余种，广布于世界各地。裸子植物形成种子时不形成子房和果实，胚珠和种子是裸露的，由此而得名裸子植物。

（1）银杏科 Ginkgoaceae

银杏 *Ginkgo biloba* L.

（2）松科 Pinaceae

红松 *Pinus koraiensis* Sieb.

（3）红豆杉科 Taxaceae

东北红豆杉 *Taxus cuspidata* Sieb. Et. Zucc.

（4）麻黄科 Ephedraceae

麻黄 *Ephedra sinica* Stapf.

（三）被子植物　**Angiospermae**

被子植物是植物界进化最高级、种类最多、分布最广的类群。现知被子植物有 1 万多属，20 多万种，占植物界的一半。我国有 2700 多属，约 3 万种，是药用植物最多的类群。和裸子植物相比，被子植物有真正的花，故又叫有花植物；胚珠包藏在子房内，得到良好的保护，子房在受精后形成的果实，既保护种子又以各种方式帮助种子散布。

1. 双子叶植物纲　Dicotyledoneae

＊（1）蓼科 Polygonaceae　多为草本。茎节常膨大。单叶互生，托叶膜质，包围茎节基部成托叶鞘。花多两性，辐射对称，排成穗状、圆锥状或头状花序，花被片 3 ~ 6，常花瓣状，分离或基部合生，宿存；雄蕊 3 ~ 9；子房上位，由 3（稀 2 或 4）心皮合生组成，1 室，1 胚珠，基生胎座。瘦果凸镜形、三棱形或近圆形，包于宿存花被内。种子有胚乳。染色体：X = 7 ~ 20。

约 30 属，800 余种，主要分布于北温带。我国 14 属，200 多种，全国均有分布。已知药用 8 属，约 123 种。

本科突出特征：草本，有膜质托叶鞘。花单被，子房上位。瘦果包于宿存花被内。

何首乌 *Polygonum multiflorum* Thunb.

波叶大黄 *Rheum undulatum* Auct.

圆叶大黄 *R. Rhaponticum* L.

*（2）毛茛科　Ranunculaceae　草本，稀木质藤本。叶互生或基生，少对生，如铁线莲属（Clematis），单叶或复叶，无托叶。花通常两性，辐射对称或两侧对称，如乌头属（Aconitum），花单生或排成聚伞花序、总状花序；萼片3至多数，雄蕊和心皮多数，离生，螺旋状排列，稀定数，子房上位，1室，每心皮含1至多数胚珠。聚合蓇葖果或聚合瘦果，稀浆果，如类叶升麻属（Actaea）。

约50属，2000种，主要分布于北温带。我国有42种，800余种，全国各地均有分布，已知药用的有30属，近500种。

本科突出特征：草本，叶分裂或复叶。花两性，雄蕊和雌蕊常为多数，离生。螺旋状排列在膨大的花托上；多为聚合瘦果。

乌头 *Aconitum carmichaeli* Debx.

黄花乌头 *A. coreanum*（Levl.）Rap.

北乌头 *A . kusnezoffii* Rechb.

升麻 *Cimicifuga dahurica* Maxim.

棉团铁线莲 *Clematis hexapetala* Pall.

东北铁线莲 *C. mandshurica* Rupr.

白头翁 *Pulsatilla chinensis*（Bge.）Rgl.

毛茛 *Ranunculus japonicus* Thunb.

唐松草 *Thalictrum minus* L.

三颗针 *Berberis julianae* Schneid.

芍药 *Paeonia lactiflora* Pall.

牡丹 *P. suffruticosa* Andr.

（3）马兜铃科 Aristolochiaceae

细辛 *Aristolochia heterotropoides*（Maxim.）Kitag.

（4）罂粟科 Papaveraceae

东北延胡索 *Corydalis ambigua* Cham. et Schltd.

齿瓣延胡索 *Corydalis turtschaninovii* Bess.

白屈菜 *Chelidonium majus* L.

*（5）十字花科　Cruciferae　一年生或多年生草本，植物体有的含辛辣液汁。单叶互生；无托叶。花两性，辐射对称，多排成总状或圆锥花序；萼片4，排成2轮；花瓣4，十字形排列；雄蕊6，4长2短，称四强雄蕊；子房上位，2心皮组成，由假隔膜隔成2室，侧膜胎座，胚珠1至多数。长角果或短角果，多2瓣开裂。种子无胚乳。

本科植物约350属，3200种，广布世界各地，主产北温带。我国有96属，约430种。已知药用75种，分布于全国各地。

本科突出特征：叶互生，无托叶，萼片4，排成2轮，花瓣4，十字形排列，四强雄蕊。长角果或短角果。

菘蓝 *Isatis indigotica* Auct.

*（6）蔷薇科　Rosaceae　草本，灌木或乔木。常具刺。单叶或复叶，多互生，通常有托叶，托叶有时早落或附生于叶柄。花两性，辐射对称；单生或排成伞房或圆锥

花序；花托凸起或凹陷，花被与雄蕊合成一碟状、坛状或壶状的花筒（hypanthium），萼片、花瓣和雄蕊均着生花筒的边缘；萼片5，花瓣5，分离，稀无瓣（地榆属 Sanguisorba）；雄蕊通常多数；心皮1至多数，分离或结合，子房上位至下位，每室1至多数胚珠。蓇葖果、瘦果、核果或梨果。

约124属，3300余种，分布于全世界。我国约有48属，900余种，广布全国各地。已知药用约43属，363种。

本科突出特征：叶互生，有托叶。花两性，5基数，轮状排列，通常具杯形、盘形或壶形的花筒，形成周位花。种子无胚乳。

龙牙草 *Agrimonia pilosa* Ledeb.

山里红 *Crataegua pinnatifida* var. *major* Br.

山杏 *Prunus ansu*（Maxim.）Kom.

地榆 *Sanguisorba officinalis* L.

珍珠梅 *Sorbaria sorbifolia*（L.）A. Br.

＊（7）豆科 Leguminosae 木本或草本，有时藤本。叶互生，多为复叶，有托叶。花序各种；花两性，辐射对称或两侧对称；萼5裂，花瓣5，通常分离，多数为蝶形花；雄蕊10，二体，少数分离或下部合生；心皮1，子房上位，胚珠1至多数，边缘胎座。荚果。种子无胚乳。

约700属，17000种，广布世界各地。是种子植物第三大科，仅次于菊科和兰科。我国包括引种的共约160属，1300余种。全国各地均有分布。已知药用109属，600多种。

本科突出特征：多为复叶，有托叶；蝶形花或假蝶形花，单心皮雌蕊，二体雄蕊。荚果。

甘草 *Glycyrrhiza uralensis* Fisch.

东北黄芪 *Astragalus membranaceus* Bge.

白扁豆 *Dolichos lablab* L.

苦参 *Sophora flavescens* Ait.

蒙古黄芪 *A. membranaceus* var. *mongholicus*（Bge.）Hsiao.

（8）大戟科 Euphorbiaceae

巴豆 *Croton tiglium* L.

狼毒 *Euphorbia fischeriana* Steudel.

（9）芸香科 Rutaceae

白鲜 *Dictamnus dasycarpus* Turcz.

黄柏 *Phellodendron amurense* Rupr.

＊（10）五加科 Araliaceae 木本，稀多年生草本。茎常有刺。叶多互生，常为掌状复叶或羽状复叶，少为单叶。花小，两性，稀单性，辐射对称；伞形花序或集成头状花序，常排成总状或圆锥状；萼齿5，小形，花瓣5~10，分离；雄蕊5~10，生于花盘边缘；子房下位，由2~15心皮合生，通常2~15室，每室1胚珠。浆果或核果。

80属，900多种，广布于热带和温带。我国有23属，172种，除新疆外，几乎全国均有分布。已知药用 18 属，112 种，多有驱风利湿，舒经活血或益气健脾，补肾安神的功效。

本科突出特征：多木本，伞形花序，5 基数花，子房下位，每室 1 胚珠。多为浆果。

刺五加 *Acanthopanax senticosus*（Rupr. et Maxim.）Harms.

辽东楤木 *Aralia elata*（Miq.）Seem.

人参 *Panax ginseng* C. A. May

*（11）伞形科 Umbelliferea 草本，常含挥发油。茎常中空，有纵棱。叶互生，叶片分裂或为复叶，稀为单叶；叶柄基部扩大成鞘状。花小，两性，多为复伞形花序，稀为单伞形花序；复伞形花序基部具总苞片或缺；花萼和子房贴生，萼齿 5 或不明显；花瓣 5；雄蕊 5；子房下位，由 2 心皮合生，2 室，每室有一胚珠。双悬果；每分果外面有 5 条棱。

约 275 属，2900 种，广布于北温带、亚热带和热带。我国有 95 属，540 种，全国均产。已知药用 55 属，234 种。

本科突出特征：芳香本草，有鞘状叶柄，花五基数，子房下位，两室，具上位花盘（花柱基），多为复伞形花序。双悬果。

白芷 *Angelica anomala* Lallem.

独活 *A. dahurica* Benth. et Hook.

柴胡 *Bupleurum chinensis* DC.

大叶柴胡 *B. longiradiatum* Turcz.

小茴香 *Foeniculum vulgare* Mill.

川芎 *Ligusticum wallichii* Franch.

防风 *Saposhnikovia divaricata*（Turcz.）Schischk.

北沙参 *Glehnia littoralis*（A. Gray）Fr. Schmidt.

（12）夹竹桃科 Apocynaceae

罗布麻 *Apocynum venetum* L.

长春花 *Catharanthus roseus*（L.）G. Don.

夹竹桃 *Nerium indicum* Mill.

（13）萝摩科 Asclepiadaceae

杠柳 *Periploca sepium* Bunge.

（14）紫草科 Bolemoniaceae

黄花夹竹桃 *Thevetia peruviana*（Pers.）K. Schum.

紫草 *Lithospermum erythrorhizon* Sieb. et Zucc.

*（15）唇形科 Labiatae 常为草本，多含挥发油。茎四方形，叶对生。花序通常为腋生聚伞花序排成轮伞花序；花两性。两侧对称；花萼 5 裂，唇形；雄蕊 4，2 强，花盘常存在；雌蕊由 2 个心皮组成，子房上位，通常 4 深裂形成假 4 室，每室有 1 颗胚珠，花柱着生于 4 裂子房的底部。果实为 4 枚小坚果。

约 220 属，3500 种，全球广布，主产地为地中海及中亚地区。我国约 99 属，808

种，全国均产。国产种类中，已知药用75属，436种。

本科突出特征：草本，具芳香气。茎方形。叶对生。轮伞花序；花冠二唇形，子房深4裂，花柱着生于4裂子房的底部。4枚小坚果。

益母草 *Leonurus japonicus* Houtt.

薄荷 *Mentha haplocalyx* Brig.

紫苏 *Perilla nankinensis*（Lour.）Decne.

夏枯草 *Prunella asiatica* Nakai.

丹参 *Salvia miltiorhiza* Bge.

黄芩 *Scutellaria baicalensis* Georgi.

*（16）茄科 Solanaceae 草本或木本。叶常互生，无托叶。花单生、簇生或成各种花序；两性，辐射对称；花萼常5裂，宿存，果时常增大；花冠合瓣成钟状、漏斗状、辐状，裂片5；雄蕊常5枚，着生在花冠上；子房上位，由2心皮合成，2室，中轴胎座，胚珠常多数。浆果或蒴果。

本科突出特征：叶互生。花辐射对称，5基数，子房2室，胚珠多数。花萼常5裂，宿存，茎具双韧维管束。

颠茄 *Atropa belladonna* L.

白花曼陀罗 *Datura metel* L.

莨菪 *Hyoscyamus niger* L.

枸杞 *Lycium chinense* Mill.

龙葵 *Solanum nigrum* L.

（17）玄参科 Scrophulariaceae

地黄 *Rehmannia glutinosa* Libosch.

玄参 *Scrophularia ningpoensis* Hemsl.

（18）忍冬科 Caprifoliaceae

金银花 *Lonicera japonica* Thunb.

（19）败酱科 Valerianaceae

黄花败酱 *Patrinia scabiosaefolia* Fisch. et Trev.

（20）桔梗科 Campanulaceae

轮叶沙参 *Adenophora tetraphylla* Fisch.

心叶沙参 *A. tracheloides* Maxim.

党参 *Codonopsis pilosula*（Franch.）Nannf.

桔梗 *Platycodon grandiflorus*（Jacq.）DC.

*（21）菊科 Compositae 常为草本，稀木本。有的具乳汁或树脂道。单叶，互生，无托叶；花密集成头状花序，下围以总苞。头状花序有时可再集成总状、伞房状等复花序。花两性，稀单性或中性；分为管状花，舌状花二型，有同型的（全为管状花或舌状花），有异型的（外围为舌状花，中央为管状花）；萼片常变成冠毛，雄蕊常5枚，为聚药雄蕊，花丝分离，着生花冠管上，花药合生成管状；雌蕊由2心皮合生，1室，子房下位，具1倒生胚珠，柱头2裂。连萼瘦果（与瘦果的区别在于有花托或萼

管参与果实形成）。染色体：X = 8、9、10、12、15、16、17。

本科突出特征：头状花序具总苞，有舌状花或管状花，聚药雄蕊，子房下位，1室，具1胚珠。连萼瘦果。

菊科是被子植物第一大科，约1000属，25000 ~ 30000 种，占有花植物的 1/10，全球广布，主产温带地区。我国约227属，2323 种，全国广布，已知药用155属，778种，占我国菊科植物的近 1/3。

青蒿 *Artemisia apiacea* Hance.

紫菀 *Aster tataricus* L.

关苍术 *A. japonica* Koidz. ex Kitam.

朝鲜苍术 *A. koreana*（Nakai.）Kitam.

白术 *A. macrocephala* Koidz.

红花 *Carthamus tinctorius* L.

野菊花 *Chrysanthemum indicum* L.

北苍术 *Atractylodes chinensis*（Bunge.）Koidz.

2. 单子叶植物纲　Monocotyledoneae

*（1）百合科 Liliaceae　多为多年生草本，具鳞茎或根状茎，少数为灌木。单叶，互生或基生，少数对生或轮生极少数退化成鳞片状，茎扁化成叶状枝（如天门冬属、假叶树属）。花序种种；花常两性，辐射对称；花被片6，花瓣状，2轮排列，分离或合生；雄蕊6；子房上位，3心皮合生成3室，中轴胎座，胚珠常多数。蒴果或浆果。染色体：X = 3 ~ 27。

233 属，约4000 种，广布全球，以温带及亚热带地区为多。我国有60属，570 种（包括引进栽培的属和种），分布南北各地，西南地区最丰富。已知药用46属，358 种。

本科突出特征：为典型的 3 数花，雄蕊 6，子房上位，3 心皮，中轴胎座，3 室；常具鳞茎、根状茎。

芦荟 *Aloe vera* L. var. *chinensis*（Haw.）Breg.

知母 *Anemarrhena asphodeloides* Bunge.

铃兰 *Convallaria beiskei* Miq.

平贝母 *Fritillaria ussuriensis* Maxim.

黄花菜 *Hemerocallis minor* Mill.

卷丹 *Lilium lancifolium* Thunb.

细叶百合 *L. pumilum* DC.

麦冬 *Ophipopgon japonicus*（L. F.）Kor – Gawl.

玉竹 *Polygonatum odoratum* Mill. Druce.

藜芦 *Veratrum nigrum* L.

（2）薯蓣科 Dioscoreaceae

山药 *Dioscorea batatas* Decne .

穿山龙 *D. nipponica* Makino.

（3）禾本科 Gramineae

薏苡 *Coix lacryma – jobi* L.

（4）天南星科 Araceae

石菖蒲 *Acorus gramineus* Soland.

东北天南星 *Arisaema amurense* Maxim.

掌叶半夏 *Pinellia pedatisecta* Schott.

（5）姜科 Zingiberaceae

砂仁 *Amomun villosum* Lour.

（6）兰科 Orchidaceae

天麻 *Gastrodia elata* Bl.

二、标本室实习

观察和重点掌握下列生药的性状：冬虫夏草、茯苓、昆布、海藻、海人草、猪苓、麦角、绵马贯众、石韦、海金沙、麻黄、大黄、何首乌、川乌、附子、黄连、白芍、牡丹皮、厚朴、五味子、延胡索、阿片、大青叶、板蓝根、苦杏仁、山楂、仙鹤草（鹤草芽）、黄芪、甘草、苦参、番泻叶、毒扁豆、黄柏、枳实、毛果云香叶、人参、三七、刺五加、柴胡、当归、川芎、小茴香、独活、白芷、毒毛旋花子、香加皮 、黄芩、薄荷、丹参、益母草、颠茄草、洋金花、枸杞子、洋地黄叶、地黄、毛花地黄叶、白术、苍术、红花、青蒿、除虫菊、茵蒿花、半夏、天南星、川贝母、浙贝母、铃兰、大蒜、天麻、地龙、水蛭、斑蝥、蟾酥、熊胆、麝香、牛黄、羚羊角、朱砂、石膏、砒石。

Experiment 20　Practicing in Medicinal Plant Garden and Herbarium

Aim

1. Comprehend the plant classification through morphous observation of plants, especially in aspect of flower properties.

2. Understand 30 kinds of typical plants belonged to different families, remember their main morphological characteristics, comprehend the concept of family more deeply, and learn the morphologic characteristics of ten families.

3. Grasp the morphologic characteristics and identification methods of the emphasized crude drugs through the practice in the herbarium.

Methods

1. Practice in medicinal plant garden

Divide students into two groups, be familiar with plants morphous under the guidance of a teacher, and take the observation note and write down the comprehension of plants classification. The point is to observe the plant morphous of the main families※.

（1）Pteridophyta　There are vascular tissues in pteridophyta, but it is lowclass in the higher plant with the obvious alternation of generations; sporophyte and gametophyte may independently live and sporophyte is developed. It is terrestrial, parasitic or aquatic. The common frond (sporophyte) is differentiated into root, stem and leaf. Adventitious root are common; rhizome are usually coated with hair or scale; leaves, which are divided into macrophyll and microphyll according to their origin and morphological characteristics, mostly developped from rhizome. Sporangium is single or aggregated to form sporangium mass distributed on the backside or verge of rotundity or fringy sporophyll. Most sporangia gather to form variform spike, with or without indusium. Spores are mostly homomorphic, and less are hetromorphic, which are generate in megasporangium and microsporangium respectively.

About 12 000 species Pteridophyta plants are distributed over world, especially in tropics and subtropics, mostly as herbaceous plants. There are about 2600 species in our country and 455 species are used as medicinal plants.

Stlaginellaceae: *Selaginella tamariscina* (Beauv) Spr.

Equisetaceae: *Equisetum arvense* L., *E. hyemale* (L.) Boern.

Dryopteridacea: *Cyrtomium fortonei* J. Sm.; *Dryopteris crassirhizoma* Nakai.

Polypodiaceae: *Pyrrosia petiolosa* (Christ) Ching

(2) Gymnospermae   Most sporophytes are developed evergreen woody. Their taproot is developed, which possesses cambium and cork cambium to carry out the secondary growth. The vascular bundles arrange annularly, most of xylem are tracheids, and sieve cells without companion cells in phloem. Gametophyte is tiny and very degenerate, completely parasitizing in sporophyte. Water as a medium is not necessary in the fertilization of sperm in male gametophyte with ootid in female gametophyte. Its flowers always lack perianth and ovules are naked.

In ancient, Gymnosperm and Pteridophyte were distributed all over the world, later they were degraded and most of them were extinct. Now, only 12 families, 71 genera and about 800 species are existent. There are 11 families, 41 genera and 236 species in our country and 10 families, 25 genera and about 100 species are belong to medicinal plants. When gymnosperm seed is produced, no germen or fruit is formed and its ovule and seed are naked, so it is named Gymnosperm.

Ginkgoaceae: *Ginkgo biloba* L.

Pinaceae: *Pinus koraiensis* Sieb.

Taxaceae: *Taxus cuspidata* Sieb. et. Zucc.

Ephedraceae: *Ephedra sinica* Stapf.

(3) Angiospermae   It is the most advanced plants with the greatest diversities and the most extensive distribution in vegetation kingdom. There are more than 10 000 known genera and 200 000 species, accounting for half of plants in vegetable kingdom. There are more than 2700 genera and about 30 000 species in our country. It is the largest group in medicinal plants. Compared with Gymnosperm, Angiosperm possesses true flower, hence it is named flowering plants or anthophytes; ovule enclosed by ovary is protected well, ovary forms fruit after

fertilization, not only protects seed but assists seed dispersal by the various ways.

①Dicotyledoneae

* Ⅰ. Polygonaceae

Habit: mostly herb, usually with swollen nodes.

Leaves: alternate, simple, membranaceous ocrea to surround the base of petiole.

Flowers: usually bisexual, actinomorphic; spike, panicle or capitulum; 3 – 6 choripetalous or basal synpetalous and indeciduous petaloid perianthes; 3 – 9 stamens; superior ovary composed by 3 (seldom 2 or 4) united carpels with 1 locule and 1 ovule inside, basal placentation.

Fruit: burning glass, triangle – edged like or rotund achene enclosed in indeciduous perianth.

Seeds: containing abundant endosperm.

Chromosome: X = 7 – 20.

There are about 30 genera and 800 species in the family, mainly distributed in northern-temperate zone. 14 genera and more than 200 species are in our country.

Outstanding characteristics: herb; membranaceous ocrea; monochlamydeous; superior ovary; achene enclosed in indeciduous perianth.

Polygonum multiflorum Thunb.

Rheum undulatum Auct.

R. rhaponticum L.

* Ⅱ. Ranunculaceae

Habit: herb, unusual woody vine.

Leaves: alternate or basal, scarcely opposite, such as Clematis; simple and compound exstipulate leaf.

Flowers: typically bisexual, actinomorphic or zygomorphic, as Aconitum; solitary, cymes or racemes; Calyx with 3 or many sepals; corolla with 3 or many petals, rarely without petal; many spirally arranged adelphia and distinct carpels; superior ovary, 1 locule, 1 or many ovules in locule.

Fruit: aggregate follicle or aggregate achene, rarely berry, as Actaea.

There are about 50 genera and 2 000 species in the family, mainly distributed in northern-temperate zone. 42 genera and 800 species are throughout in our country.

Outstanding characteristics: herb; divided or compound leaf; bisexual flowers; many adelphia and distinct carpels spirally arranged on inflated receptacle; mostly aggregate achene.

Aconitum carmichaeli Debx.

A. coreanum (Levl.) Rap.

A. kusnezoffii Rechb.

Cimicifuga dahurica Maxim.

Clematis hexapetala Pall.

C. mandshurica Rupr.

Pulsatilla chinensis (Bge.) Rgl.

Ranunculus japonicus Thunb.

Thalictrum minus L.

Berberis julianae Schneid.

Paeonia lactiflora Pall.

P. suffruticosa Andr.

Ⅲ. Aristolochiaceae

Aristolochia heterotropoides (Maxim.) Kitag.

Ⅳ. Papaveraceae

Corydalis ambigua Cham. et Schltd.

Corydalis turtschaninovii Bess.

Chelidonium majus L.

* Ⅴ. Crucifereae

Habit: annual or perennial herb with pungent juice.

Leaves: simple, alternate, stipules absent.

Flowers: bisexual, actinomorphic; raceme orpanicle; calyx with 4 sepals arranged in 2 whorles; corolla with 4 petals arranged in cruciform; 6 stamens, in which 4 long and 2 short, hence called tetradynamous stamen; gynoecium with 2 carpels divided into 2 locules by false dissepiment, superior overy, parietal placenta, 1 or many ovules.

Fruit: silique or silicle.

There are about 350 genera and 3 200 species in the family, distributed throughout the world, mainly in northerntemperate zone. About 96 genera and 430 species are distributed throughout our country, 75 species belong to medicinal plants.

Outstanding characteristics: alternate leaves, exstipulate; calyx with 4 sepals arranged in 2 whorles; corolla with 4 petals arranged in cruciform; tetradynamous stamen; silique or silicle.

Isatis indigotica Auct.

* Ⅵ. Rosaceae

Habit: herb, shrub or tree, usually with thorns.

Leaves: alternate, simple or compound, with paired stipules that are sometimescaducous or adnascent to the petiole.

Flowers: bisexual, actinomorphic, solitary, corymb or panicle; protuberant or invaginated receptacle; patelloid, urceolar or pot – shaped flower tube (hypanthium) formed by perianth and stamen, petals and stamens attach along rim of tube, ; calyx with 5 sepals, 5 separated petals or rarely absent (Sanguisorba) ; numerous stamens; 1 or many separated or united carpels, superior or inferior ovary; 1 or more ovules in per carpel.

Fruit: achene, follicle, pome or drupe.

There are about 124 genera and 3, 300 species in the family, distributed throughout the world. 48 genera and about 900 species are distributed throughout our country, in which about 43 genera and 363 species belong to medicinal plants.

Outstanding characteristics: alternate leaf with stipule; bisexual rotiform arranging flowers, perigynous flowers usually formed by patelloid, urceolar or pot – shaped flower tuber and exendospermous seed.

Agrimonia pilosa Ledeb.

Crataegua pinnatifida var. *major* Br.

Prunus ansu (Maxim.) Kom.

Sanguisorba officinalis L.

Sorbaria sorbifolia (L.) A. Br.

∗ Ⅶ. Leguminosae

Habit: wood or herb, sometimes vine.

Leaves: mostly alternate compound leaf with stipule.

Flowers: various inflorescence; bisexual, actinomorphic or zygomorphic; calyx with 5 lobes, corolla with 5 separated petals, mostly papillionaceous flower; 10 stamens, mostly diadelphous stamens, a few separated or inferior part confluent stamen; 1 carpel, superior overy, 1 or many ovules and marginal placenta.

Fruit: Legume.

Seed: Exendospermous.

There are about 700 genera and 17 000 species in the family, distributed throughout the world. It is the third large family in spermatophyte, second only compositae and orchidaceae. 160 genera and 1300 species are distributed allover our country, in which 109 genera and more than 600 species are belong to medicinal plants.

Outstanding characteristics: mostly leaves are compound and possess stipule; papillionaceous or pseudo – papillionaceous flower; simple pistil; legume.

Glycyrrhiza uralensis Fisch.

Astragalus membranaceus Bge.

Dolichos lablab L.

Sophora flavescens Ait.

A. menbranaceus var. *mongholicus* (Bge.) Hsiav.

Ⅷ. Euphoubiaceae

Croton tiglium L.

Euphorbia fischeriana Steudel.

Ⅸ. Rutaceae

Dictamnus dasycarpus Turcz.

Phellodendron amurense Rupr.

* X. Araliaceae

Habit: wood, rarely perennial herb, with thorns on stem.

Leaves: alternate, palmately or pinnately compound leaf, rarely simple leaf.

Flowers: small, bisexual, rarely unisexual, actinomorphic; umbel or capitulum arranged in compound raceme or panicle; small calyx with 5 dentes; corolla with 5 – 10 petals; 5 – 10 stamens attach on the brim of floral disc; inferior ovary, gynoecium formed by 2 – 15 fused carpels, usually 2 – 15 locules, 1 ovule in each locule.

Fruit: berry or drupe.

There are 80 genera and more than 900 species in the family, distributed in tropics and temperate zone. 23 genera and 172 species are widely distributed in our country except Xin-Jiang. 18 genera and 112 species belong to medicinal plants with the effects of dispelling wind and dampness, promoting meridian and blood flow, or nourishing Qi to invigorate spleen, tonifying kidney to relieve mental strain.

Outstanding characteristics: mostly wood; umbel; inferior ovary; 1 ovule in each locule; mostly berry.

Acanthopanax senticosus (Rupr. et Maxim.) Harms.

Aralia elata (Miq.) Seem.

Panax ginseng C. A. May

* XI. Umbelliferea

Habit: herb, hollow stem withlongitudinal arrises, contained aromatic oil.

Leaves: alternate, divided leaf blade or compound leaf with sheath at the base of petiole.

Flowers: Bisexual, small; compound umbel, rarely simple umbel; involucre at the base of compound umbel or absence; calyx adnated to ovary with 5 dentes; 5 petals; 5 stamens; inferior ovary formed by 2 united carpels, 2 locules, 1 ovule in each locule.

Fruit: cremocarp with 5 ridges.

There are about 275 genera and 2900 species under the family, distributed in northern temperate zone, subtropical zone and tropics. 95 genera and 540 species are distributed throughout our country, in which 55 genera and 234 species belong to medicinal plants.

Outstanding characteristics: Aromatic herb with sheath at the base of petiole, 5 radix flowers, inferior ovary, 2 locules, epigynous flower disc (style base), compound umbel, cremocarp.

Angelica anomala Lallem.

A. dahurica Benth. et Hook.

Bupleurum chinensis DC.

B. longiradiatum Turcz.

Foeniculum vulgare Mill.

Ligusticum wallichii Franch.

Saposhnikovia divaricata (Turcz.) Schischk.

Glehnia littoralis (A. Gray) Fr. Schmidt.

Ⅻ. Apocynaceae

Apocynum venetum L.

Catharanthus roseus (*L.*) *G. Don.*

Nerium indicum *Mill.*

Ⅻ. Asclepiadaceae

Periploca sepium Bunge.

ⅩⅣ. Bolemoniaceae

Thevetia peruviana (*Pers.*) K. Schum

Lithospermum erythrorhizon *Sieb. et* Zucc

* ⅩⅤ. Labiatae

Habit: usually herb with square stem, contained aromatic oil.

Leaves: opposite.

Flowers: bisexual, zygomorphic, verticillaster arranged by axillary cyme; calyx with 5 lobes, labiate corolla, 4 stamens, didynamous stamen; gynoecium united by 2 carpels, superior ovary usually splits deeply into falsely 4 – locular, 1 ovule in each false locule, style on base of ovary.

Fruit: 4 nutlets.

There are about 220 genera and 3500 species under the family, distributed throughout the world, mainly inthe Mediterranean and central Asia. 99 genera and 808 species are throughout our country, in which 75 genera and 436 species belong to medicinal plants.

Outstanding characteristics: aromatic herb with square stem; opposite leaf; verticillaster; ovary splits deeply into falsely 4 – locular, style attached to base of ovary; 4 nutlets.

Leonurus japonicus Houtt.

Mentha haplocalyx Brig.

Perilla nankinensis (Lour.) Decne.

Prunella asiatica Nakai.

Salvia miltiorhiza Bge.

Scutellaria baicalensis Georgi.

ⅩⅥ. Solanaceae

Habit: herb or wood.

Leaves: alternate, exstipulate.

Flowers: bisexual, actinomorphic; single, cluster or various of inflorescences; persistent calyx with 5 lobes, swollened during fruiting period; synpetalous corolla with 5 sepals to form mitriform, funnel – shaped, radiat; 5 stamens inserted on the corolla tube; gynoecium formed by 2 carpels, superior ovary with 2 locules, axile placenta and numerous ovules.

Fruit: berry or capsule.

Outstanding characteristics: alternate leaf, 5 radix actinomorphic flower, ovary 2 locules, numerous ovules; persistent calyx with 5 lobes, bicollateral bundles in stem.

Atropa belladonna L.

Datura metel L.

Hyoscyamusniger L.

Lycium chinense Mill.

Solanum nigrum L.

XVII. Scrophulariaceae

Rehmannia glutinosa Libosch.

Scrophularia ningpoensis Hemsl.

XVIII. Caprifoliaceae

Lonicera japonica Thunb.

XIX. Valerianaceae

Patrinia scabiosaefolia Fisch. et Trev.

XX. Campanulaceae

Adenophora tetraphylla Fisch.

A. tracheloides Maxim.

Codonopsis pilosula (Franch.) Nannf.

Platycodon grandiflorus (Jacq.) DC.

* XXI. Compositae

Habit: herb usually with latex or resin canal.

Leaves: simple, alternate, exstipulate.

Flowers: capitulum gathered by florets, surrounded inferior part by involucre, raceme or cyme sometimes formed by capitulum; bisexual, rarely monosexual or neutral; ligulate or tuberlar corolla with 5 petals, calyx represented by pappus; 5 stamens, syngenesious stamen, separated capillament inserts on corol tube and coadnate anther to form tube; pistil formed by 2 coadnate carpels, 1 locule, inferior ovary with 1 anatropous ovule, 2 divided chapiter.

Fruits: cypsela (receptacle and calyx tube participate the fruit – forming)

chromosome: X = 8、9、10、12、15、16、17。

This is the first big family in angiosperm, includes about 1000 genera and 25 000 – 30 000 species, 1/10 of flowering plants, distributed throughout the world, mainly in northern temperate zone. There are about 227 genera and 2 323 species all over our country, in which 155 genera and 778 species, 1/3 of plants of this family, belong to medicinal plants.

Outstanding characteristics: capitulum with involucre, ligulate or tubular flower, synantherous stamen, inferior ovary, 1 locule, 1 ovule and epiachene.

Artemisia apiacea Hance.

Aster tataricus L.

A. japonica Koidz. ex Kitam.

A. koreana （Nakai.) Kitam.

A. macrocephala Koidz.

Carthamus tinctorius L.

Chrysanthemum indicum L.

Atractylodes chinensis （Bunge.) Koidz.

②Monocotyledoneae

＊Ⅰ. Liliaceae

Habit: mostly perennial herb, with bulb or rhizome, few shrubs. In some genera, phylloclade is formed by planation.

Leaves: simple, alternate or basal, few opposite of whorled, rarely degenerated to scale – like leaf.

Flowers: various of inflorescence; usually bisexual, actinomorphic; free or united petaloid perianth with 6 sepals in 2 whorls; 6 stamens; superior ovary formed by 3 united carpels, usually 3 locules, axile placenta, numerous ovules.

Fruit: capsule or berry.

Chromosome: $X = 3 - 27$.

There are 233 genera and about 4000 species in the family, distributed throughout the world, mainly in temperate zone and subtropics. 60 genera and 570 species （including the cultural) in our country, distributed everywhere, mainly in the southwest, in which 46 genera and 358 species belong to medicinal plants.

Outstanding characteristics: 3 radix flowers, 6stamens, superior ovary, 3 carpels, axile placenta, 3 locules, bulb and rhizomes.

Aloe vera L. var. *chinensis* （Haw.) Breg.

Anemarrhena asphodeloides Bunge.

Convallaria beiskei Miq.

Fritillaria ussuriensis Maxim.

Hemerocallis minor Mill.

Lilium lancifolium Thunb.

L. pumilum DC.

Ophipopgon japonicus （L. F.) Kor – Gawl.

Polygonatum odoratum Mill. Druce.

Veratrum nigrum L.

Ⅱ. Dioscoreaceae

Dioscorea batatas Decne .

D. nipponica Makino.

Ⅲ. Gramineae

Coix lacryma – jobi L.

Ⅳ. Araceae

Acorus gramineus Soland.

Arisaema amurense Maxim.

Pinellia pedatisecta Schott.

Ⅴ. Zingiberaceae

Amomun villosum Lour.

Ⅵ. Orchidaceae

Gastrodia elata Bl.

2. Practice in the herbarium

Obtain the morphous of the crude drugs as follows:

Aweto, hoelen, sea tangle, kelp, digenea, chuling, ergot, male fern rhizome, shearer's pyrrosia leaf, Japanese climbing fern spore, ephedra, rhubar, fleeceflower root, common monkshood mother root, prepared common monkshood daughter root, golden thread, white peony alba, tree peony bark, magnolia bark, Chinese magnolivine fruit, yanhusuo, opium, dyers woad leaf, isatis root, bitter apricot seed, hawthorn fruit, hairyvein agrimonia herd (gemma agrimoniae), milkvetch root, liquorice root, lightyellow sophora root, senna leaf, calabar bean, amoorcorn tree bark, immature orange fruit, Ginseng, Sanchi, manyprickle acanthopanax root, Chinese thorowax root, Chinese angelica, Szechwan lovage rhizome, fennel, doubleteeth pubesscent angelica root, dahurian angelica root, icaja, Chinese silkvine root – bark, baical skullcap root, peppermint, motherwort herb, belladonna herb, datura flower, barbary wolfberry fruit, digitalis leaf, rehmannia root, Grecian foxglove leaves, largehead atractylodes rhizome, atractylodes rhizome, safflower, sweet wormwood herb, insect – flower, pinellia tuber, Jackinthepulpit tuber, tendrilleaf fritillary bulb, thunberg fritillary bulb, lily – of – the – valley, garlic, tall gastrodis tuber, lumbricus, leech, blister beetle, toad venom, bear gall, musk, cow – bezoar, antelope horn, cinnabar, gypsum and arsenolite ore.

附　录

一、常用显微镜试剂的配制

1. **清洁剂**　取乙醚 7 ml 和无水乙醇 3 ml 混合，装入滴瓶，备用，用于擦拭显微镜镜头上的油迹和污垢等（瓶口必须塞紧，以免挥发）。

2. **F. A. A 固定液（又称万能固定剂）**　福尔马林（38% 甲醛）5 ml，冰醋酸 5 ml，70% 乙醇 90 ml。幼嫩材料用 50% 乙醇代替 70% 乙醇，可防止材料收缩；还可以加入甘油 5 ml，以防止蒸发和材料变硬。此液兼可作为保存剂使用。

3. **稀甘油**　取甘油 33 ml，加蒸馏水稀释成 100 ml，再加樟脑一小块或液化苯酚 1 滴，即得。

稀甘油能使细胞稍透明及溶解某些水溶性细胞后含物，并使材料保持湿润和软化，常和水合氯醛试剂同用作临时封藏剂，可防止水合氯醛晶体析出。

4. **水合氯醛试剂**　取水合氯醛 50 g，加蒸馏水 15 ml，与甘油 10 ml 使其溶解，即得。本试液能迅速透入组织，使干燥而皱缩的细胞膨胀，细胞组织透明清晰，并能溶解淀粉粒、树脂、蛋白质和挥发油等。

5. **间苯二酚试液**　取间苯二酚 1 g，加 90% 乙醇 5 ml 溶解后，加甘油 5 ml，摇匀，即得。用于鉴别木质化的细胞壁，应用时先加 1~2 滴于被检物，约 1 分钟后，加盐酸 1 滴，木质化细胞壁因木质化程度不同而显红色或紫色。

6. **稀碘液**　取碘化钾 1 g 溶于 100 ml 蒸馏水中，再加碘 0.3 g，储于棕色瓶中。稀碘液可使淀粉粒显蓝色，糊粉粒显黄色。

7. **苏丹Ⅲ试液**　取苏丹Ⅲ 0.01 g，加 90% 乙醇 5 ml 溶解后，加甘油 5 ml，摇匀，储于棕色玻璃瓶中，保存期为 2 个月。本试液能使角质化和木栓化细胞壁显红色或橙红色，使脂肪油、挥发油或树脂显橙红色、红色或紫红色。

8. **钌红试液**　取 10% 醋酸钠溶液 1~2 ml，加钌红适量，使成酒红色，即得。本试液应临用时配制，可使黏液显红色。

9. **α-萘酚试液**　取 α-萘酚 1.5 g 溶于 95% 乙醇 10 ml，即得。应用时滴加本试液 1~2 分钟后，再滴加 80% 硫酸 2 滴，可使菊糖显紫色。

10. **氯化锌碘试液**　取氯化锌 20 g，溶于 85 ml 蒸馏水后，滴加碘-碘化钾溶液（碘化钾 3 g，碘 1.5 g，水 60 ml），不断振摇至饱和，至没有碘的沉淀出现为止，至棕色瓶内保存。

本试液可使纤维素细胞壁显蓝色和紫色。

11. **番红染液**　番红是一种碱性染料，可使木质化、木栓化、角质化的细胞壁及细胞核中的染色质和染色体染成红色。在植物组织制片中常与固绿配染。常用配方有下列两种。

（1）**番红水液**　取番红 0.1 g，溶于 100 ml 蒸馏水中，过滤后，即得。

（2）番红酒液　取番红 0.5 g 或 1 g，溶于 50% 乙醇 100 ml 中，过滤后，即得。

12. 固绿染液　固绿是一种酸性染料，可使纤维素的细胞壁和细胞质染成绿色。在植物组织制片中常与番红配染。常用固绿溶液，即取固绿 0.1 g，溶于 95% 乙醇 100 ml 中，过滤后使用。

13. 洗液　取工业用重铬酸钾（$K_2Cr_2O_7$）8 ~ 10 g 于 100 ml 清水中，加热使溶解，待冷却后，慢慢加入工业用浓硫酸（H_2SO_4）100 ml，即得。储藏于玻璃容器中。

14. IAA（0.5 mg/ml）　取 50 mg IAA 粉末，先用少量 95% 乙醇使之充分溶解，再加蒸馏水定容至 100 ml。

15. 2，4 – D　先用少量 1 mol/L 的 NaOH 溶液充分溶解，然后缓慢加入蒸馏水定容至需要体积。

16. 细胞分裂素类　KT 和 BA 等细胞分裂素类物质均溶于稀盐酸，应先用少量 1mol/L 的 HCl 溶解后再稀释至需要浓度。

17. 赤霉素　赤霉素的水溶液稳定性较差，一般用 95% 的乙醇配制成 5 ~ 10 mg/ml 的母液低温保存，使用时再稀释。

二、常用化学成分定性反应试剂

1. **1% 三氯化铁试剂**　三氯化铁 1 g，加蒸馏水使溶解成 100 ml。

2. **1% 醋酸镁甲醇液**　醋酸镁 1 g，加甲醇 100 ml。

3. **1% 三氯化铝乙醇液**　三氯化铝 1 g，溶解于 100 ml 乙醇中。

4. **0.9% 氯化钠溶液**　氯化钠 0.9 g，加水 100 ml。

5. **1.8% 氯化钠溶液**　氯化钠 1.8 g，加水 100 ml。

6. **2% 红细胞生理盐水混悬液**　兔血 10 ml，放在盛有玻璃珠的三角烧瓶中，振摇 10 分钟，除去纤维蛋白，把脱纤维血倒在离心管中，加生理盐水混匀后，离心，使血细胞下沉，反复 2 ~ 3 次，至生理盐水不再显红色，取以上红细胞 2 ml，加生理盐水 100 ml，稀释成 2% 的红细胞混悬液（本液须置冰箱保存，存期 2 ~ 3 天）。

7. **15% 三氯化铁 – 冰醋酸溶液**　1% 三氯化铁溶液 0.5 ml，加冰醋酸 100 ml。

8. **醋酸铅试液**　取醋酸铅 9.5 g，加新煮沸过的冷蒸馏水使成 100 ml。

9. **碱式醋酸铅试液**　取一氧化铅 14 g，加水 10 ml 研成糊状，用水 10 ml 洗入玻璃瓶中，加醋酸铅溶液（醋酸铅 22 g，加蒸馏水 70 ml 制成）70 ml，用力振摇 5 分钟后，时时振摇，放置 7 天，滤过，加新沸过的冷蒸馏水，使成 100 ml。

10. **稀醋酸**　冰醋酸 18 ml，加水稀释至 300 ml。

11. **2% 的 3，5 – 二硝基苯甲酸试液（Kedde 试剂）**　2% 3，5 – 二硝基苯甲酸溶液 1 ml，氢氧化钠（钾）乙醇液 3 ml 及蒸馏水 7 ml 混匀。临用时配制。

12. **1mol/L 盐酸羟胺甲醇液**　盐酸羟胺 6.95 g，加甲醇 100 ml（新鲜配制）。

13. **1mol/L 氢氧化钾甲醇试液**　取 6.2 g 氢氧化钾溶于 100 ml 甲醇中即得。

14. **1% 三氯化铁乙醇液**　三氯化铁 1 g，加乙醇使溶解成 100 ml。

15. **碘化铋钾试剂（Dragondorff 试剂）**
甲液：次硝酸铋 0.85 g，溶解于蒸馏水 40 ml、冰醋酸 10 ml 的混合液中。

乙液：碘化钾 8 g，溶解于 20 ml 水中（分别贮于棕色瓶内）。

作沉淀试剂：使用前将甲、乙两液等量混合。

作喷雾试剂：甲乙液各 5 ml 与醋酸 20 ml 及水 100 ml 混合。

16. 碘化汞钾试剂（Magner 试剂） 二氯化汞 3.4 g，溶解于 150 ml 水中；碘化钾 12.5 g，溶解于 25 ml 水中；然后将两液混合摇匀，再加水稀释至 250 ml。

17. 硅钨酸试剂（Bentrad 试剂） 硅钨酸钠 5 g，溶于 100 ml 水中，加盐酸少量至 pH 2 左右。

18. 磷钼酸试剂（Sonnenschein 试剂） 磷钼酸钠 10 g，溶于 100 ml 乙醇中。

19. 2% 茚三酮试剂 茚三酮 0.2 g，加乙醇溶解成 100 ml。

20. 0.5% 硫酸铜试液 硫酸铜 10 g，加水 100 ml。

21. 5% α−萘酚试液 取 α−萘酚 5 g，加乙醇 100 ml 溶解，即得。如不澄清，可滤过，装棕色瓶备用。

参考文献

1. 蔡少青，秦路平．生药学[M].7 版．北京：人民卫生出版社，2016.

2. 崔征．生药学[M]．北京：人民卫生出版社，2005.

3. 郑俊华．生药学实验指导[M]．北京：北京医科大学出版社，2001.

4. 国家药典委员会主编．中华人民共和国药典（一部）．2015 版［M］．北京：中国医药科技出版社，2015.

5. 徐国钧．中药材粉末显微鉴定[M]．北京：人民卫生出版社，1986.

6. 稻垣勳他．生药学实验指针[M]．南江堂．1977.

7. 孙启时．药用植物学[M]．北京：人民卫生出版社，2007.

8. 吴立军．天然药物化学[M].6 版．北京：人民卫生出版社，2011.

9. 黄璐琦．分子生药学[M].2 版．北京：北京医科大学出版社，2006.

10. V. E. Tyler, L. R. Brady, and J. E. Robbers. Pharmacognosy[M]. Ninth Edition. Philadelphia：Lea & Febiger, 1988.

11. 杨敬芝，李建北，张东明，等．中药川芎 HPLC 指纹图谱分析方法的研究[J]．药品评价，2004（04）：283 - 286.

12. 黄璐琦，胡之璧．中药鉴定新技术新方法及其应用[M]．北京：人民卫生出版社，2010.